Sports Nutrition for Women

"At last a book on sports nutrition that recognises
the needs of female exercisers."

— *Health & Fitness* magazine (UK)

Ordering

Trade bookstores in the U.S. and Canada please contact:

Publishers Group West
1700 Fourth Street, Berkeley CA 94710
Phone: (800) 788-3123   Fax: (510) 528-3444

Hunter House books are available at bulk discounts for textbook course adoptions; to qualifying community, health care, and government organizations; and for special promotions and fundraising. For details please contact:

Special Sales Department
Hunter House Inc., PO Box 2914, Alameda CA 94501-0914
Phone: (510) 865-5282   Fax: (510) 865-4295
E-mail: ordering@hunterhouse.com

Individuals can order our books from most bookstores, by calling toll-free **(800) 266-5592**, or from our website at **www.hunterhouse.com**

SPORTS NUTRITION for WOMEN

Edited by Anita Bean, B.Sc.,
and Peggy Wellington, B.Sc. (Hons), M.Phil.

First published 1995 by A & C Black (Publishers) Ltd
37 Soho Square, London W1D 3QZ
Reprinted 1996, 1998

Line diagrams on pages 49, 93, 96, and 117 by Joanna Cameron.

Hunter House Inc., Publishers
PO Box 2914
Alameda CA 94501-0914

Library of Congress Cataloging-in-Publication Data

Sports nutrition for women / edited by Anita Bean & Peggy Wellington.
      p. cm.
   Originally published: London : A&C Black Ltd, 1995.
   Includes index.
   ISBN 0-89793-351-6 (cloth) — ISBN 0-89793-350-8 (pbk.)
   1. Women athletes—Nutrition. I. Bean, Anita. II. Wellington, Peggy.
RC1218.W65 S67 2001
613.2'088'796—dc21   2001046330

Project Credits

Cover Design: Peri Poloni, Knockout Books
Book Design and Production: Jinni Fontana
Copy Editor: Kelley Blewster
Proofreader: Lee Rappold
Indexer: Kathy Talley-Jones
Acquisitions Editor: Jeanne Brondino
Associate Editor: Alexandra Mummery
Editorial and Production Assistant: Emily Tryer
Sales and Marketing Assistant: Earlita K. Chenault
Publicity Manager: Sara Long
Customer Service Manager: Christina Sverdrup
Administrator: Theresa Nelson
Computer Support: Peter Eichelberger
Publisher: Kiran S. Rana

Printed and Bound by Publishers Press, Salt Lake City, Utah
Manufactured in the United States of America

9 8 7 6 5 4 3 2 1   First Edition   01 02 03 04 05

Contents

List of Tables

List of Figures

Foreword

Nutrition is a vital part of my training schedule. I know that I must support my intensive training program with good nutritional practices; otherwise I cannot train hard and I find that I feel constantly exhausted! It's crucial that I have my diet assessed every 4 months or so, just to ensure that I am getting everything right.

I believe that all women and girls who are involved in an exercise program should be aware of the importance of sound nutrition. This book is unique in providing an ideal opportunity to evaluate common nutrition problems, to assess your own nutrition program, and to update your knowledge about the latest issues related to active women. The practical information presented here is invaluable, and the book is written in a simple-to-read style. In conclusion, this book will give most exercisers plenty to think about!

— Karen Pickering

World Champion swimmer Karen Pickering—
World Short Course Champion 1993,
double gold medallist at the
Commonwealth Games 1994,
and British record holder—
understands exactly how important
nutrition is to both performance and health.

Important Note

The material in this book is intended to provide a review of resources and information related to diet and nutrition for active women. Every effort has been made to provide accurate and dependable information. However, professionals in the field may have differing opinions, and change is always taking place. Any of the treatments described herein should be undertaken only under the guidance of a licensed health care practitioner. The author, editors, and publishers cannot be held responsible for any error, omission, professional disagreement, outdated material, or adverse outcomes that derive from use of any of the treatments or information resources in this book, either in a program of self-care or under the care of a licensed practitioner.

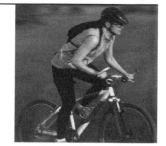

Introduction: Women, Nutrition, and Exercise

Anita Bean, B.Sc., and Peggy Wellington, B.Sc. (Hons), M.Phil.

Sports Nutrition for Women: A Practical Guide for Active Women is invaluable for all women who take exercise and sports seriously. It will enable the reader to understand the special nutritional demands placed on her body by regular exercise, and it will provide insight into the potential problems she may encounter as a result of such exercise.

A healthy diet is an essential part of all training programs, but there are a number of nutritional issues that relate specifically to women, such as bone health, iron deficiency, amenorrhea (cessation of menstrual periods), and body image. In the following pages, these issues are dealt with in depth by experts in the field of sports nutrition. In addition, active women have special nutritional needs during adolescence, pregnancy, and the later years; these are translated into practical guidelines that will help you to cope better with your training program during these times.

What special nutritional needs exist for women who play team sports? How do their requirements differ from those for athletes who participate in individual sports and fitness activities? You'll find answers to these questions in Chapter 5.

Weight management, body fat, and the problems of making weight are in the forefront of the minds of many women; indeed, weight loss or weight control are common motivations for women taking up a particular sport or exercise program in the first place. However, once the short-term weight goal has been reached (to lose a few pounds, for example), the question often arises: how far should you go? Is a lower than average body-fat level good for health and/or for sports performance? Such issues are addressed in Chapter 6, which highlights the dangers of inappropriate diets and eating patterns.

There has been some speculation that women with a tendency to eating disorders such as anorexia nervosa and bulimia nervosa are attracted to certain sports and activities that emphasize thinness or low body fat. Aesthetic concerns have become more important than health or performance for many exercising women, with the result that disordered eating patterns are now very common. This has serious health implications for women, resulting in particular in increased risk of amenorrhea, reduced fertility, and bone degeneration. Chapter 8 discusses these dangers and gives practical advice on how to recognize and treat the symptoms.

Each chapter is written by an expert in that particular field, and presents the current consensus on that topic. The science has been translated into practical advice and guidelines to enable you to put the information into practice in your own training program. References and suggestions for further reading are given at the end of most chapters.

Most important, you should be able to enjoy your sport and enjoy your food. The aim of this book is to help you achieve both—and to keep you in peak health!

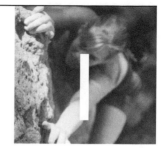

Nutritional Needs
of Active Women

Anita Bean, B.Sc.

Anita Bean, B.Sc., received the Exercise Association's 1995 Award for Special Achievement. She has a degree in nutrition and more than 10 years of experience advising sportspeople, fitness participants, and teams. Author of The Complete Guide to Sports Nutrition, *Anita has contributed to many British newspapers, magazines (including* Health & Fitness, Slimmer, *and* Exercise), *and books, and has appeared on a number of television programs. As codirector of P & A Sports Nutrition, she presents courses and seminars throughout the United Kingdom. Anita is a qualified fitness instructor and the 1991 British Bodybuilding Champion.*

Regular training places extra nutritional demands on the body, increasing energy production, altering the metabolism of carbohydrate, fat, and protein, and affecting body composition. Good nutrition is therefore of supreme importance and can help you both to improve your health and to reach your fitness goals faster. To maximize your performance and get more out of your training program, you need to fuel your body correctly and provide it with all the essential nutrients. This will help you to increase your energy levels, delay fatigue, train harder and longer, and recover more rapidly. This chapter summarizes the major nutritional needs of the body during exercise and suggests ways in which you can achieve the right balance of carbohydrate, fat, protein, vitamins, and minerals for your particular activity.

Where Does My Body's Energy Come from During Training?

Energy for training—and for living—is provided by carbohydrate, fat, and protein. These are referred to as the macronutrients, and they are the only substances in food that contain calories. The proportions of the three macronutrients used by your body depend on the type, intensity, and duration of your exercise, as well as on your fitness level and the amount of carbohydrate in your muscles before exercise.

During anaerobic types of activity (for example, sprinting, weight lifting, kicking, hitting, and jumping), carbohydrate alone is used for energy production. During aerobic activities, a mixture of carbohydrate and fat is used. If carbohydrate is in very short supply—towards the end of a long, hard training session or competition, for example—then protein will be broken down into amino acids to supply the shortfall. This may account for up to 10 percent of the fuel mixture.

The higher the training intensity, the greater the proportion of carbohydrate used and the lower the proportion of fat. For example, when running at 6 mph, about 60 percent of the fuel mixture comes from carbohydrate; when walking at 4 mph, about 40 percent of the fuel mixture comes from carbohydrate and the remainder from fat.

The longer the duration of aerobic activity, the smaller the fuel contribution from carbohydrate and the greater the contribution from fat (and, possibly, protein). Carbohydrate makes a greater contribution at the beginning of an exercise session when stores are higher; as stores gradually become depleted, it provides increasingly less of the total fuel mixture.

Beginners rely more heavily on carbohydrate for fuel at any given exercise intensity. As you become better conditioned and your aerobic fitness improves, fat is more easily broken down and accounts for a higher proportion of the fuel mixture. This is a natural adaptation to training.

What Is the Best Way to Fuel My Muscles?

For nearly all activities, the most important source of energy is carbohydrate. A low intake means low carbohydrate stores and can limit your performance, while an optimal intake can produce a significant improvement in training intensity, duration, and performance. Carbohydrate is stored as glycogen in the liver (approximately 100 grams) and muscles (approximately 300 grams) but, unfortunately, in relatively small amounts. Your glycogen stores can become depleted after 90 to 180 minutes of endurance activity, after 45 to 90 minutes of interval training, or after 30 to 45 minutes of high-intensity/anaerobic activity. The consequence of depleted glycogen is fatigue.

Starting exercise with low or suboptimal glycogen stores leads to:

- early fatigue
- reduced training intensity
- reduced training gains
- poor performance
- increased injury risk
- slower recovery
- "burnout" or overtraining syndrome (if chronic)

How Can I Speed Recovery?

Each time you exercise, you use muscle glycogen and reduce your stores, so the aim of your recovery phase is to replenish your glycogen as efficiently as possible before your next workout. You need to consider the following:

- the *amount* of carbohydrate in your diet
- the *type* of carbohydrate in your diet
- the *timing* of carbohydrate intake

How Much Carbohydrate?

At a consensus conference on sports nutrition at Lausanne, Switzerland, in 1991, scientists recommended that athletes consume at least 60 percent of energy intake from carbohydrate. This translates into 450 grams of carbohydrate for a person consuming 3,000 calories a day, or 300 grams for someone consuming 2,000 calories a day. Carbohydrates, including sugar, contain four calories per gram; protein contains 4 calories per gram; and fat contains 9 calories per gram. Knowing this, you can calculate your percentage of energy intake that should come from carbohydrate, as in the following example:

2,000 calories per day x 60 percent = 1,200 calories

1,200 calories ÷ 4 calories/gram = 300 grams carbohydrate

Calculating the percentages of calories that come from protein and fat follows the same formula; except when calculating for fat, of course, use 9 calories per gram rather than 4.

In practice, most active women need 5 to 10 grams of carbohydrate per kilogram of body weight per day depending on the intensity of their training. (To determine your body weight in kilograms, divide your body weight in pounds by 2.2.) The lower end of the range would be suitable for a woman exercising up to 1 hour per day; the upper end would be suitable for an elite athlete exercising 4 or more hours a day.

In terms of quantity of food intake, you can get 450 grams of carbohydrate from 30 bananas, 12 large potatoes, or 10 chocolate bars! Not that such a diet is advisable—this simply gives you an idea of the total amount of food that should be eaten. It is more realistic to plan your diet in 50-gram portions of carbohydrate. Examples are given below.

Portions of Food Providing About 50 Grams of Carbohydrate

- three slices of bread or toast
- one banana sandwich (two slices of bread and one banana)
- one 6-ounce baked potato with 4 ounces baked beans
- 2 ounces breakfast cereal with ½ pint low-fat milk
- 2 to 3 ounces of raisins
- two or three bananas
- 1 pint isotonic sports drink
- two or three pieces of dried fruit or small cereal bars
- seven rice cakes

- 7 ounces cooked pasta

- 6 ounces cooked rice

- one bagel

- four or five oatcakes

Which Are the Best Types of Carbohydrate?

There are two main considerations here: first, the nutritional "package" provided by the carbohydrate source; and second, the speed at which the carbohydrate is absorbed into the bloodstream.

From a nutritional point of view, the best choices are naturally occurring sources of sugars (found in fruit, vegetables, and milk) and of complex carbohydrates (found in bread, potatoes, cereals, pasta, and grains). This is because they come with a "package" of other nutrients such as vitamins, minerals, protein, and fiber (nonstarch polysaccharides).

From a performance point of view, your choice of carbohydrate depends on the timing of intake in relation to your workout. All carbohydrates are broken down into simple sugars and transported as glucose in the bloodstream, and so are equally capable of being taken up by the muscle cells and made into glycogen. As far as glycogen manufacture is concerned, then, it makes no difference whether the carbohydrate comes from processed sugar or a whole-grain food. What you need to consider is the *speed* at which the carbohydrate is converted into blood glucose and transported to the muscles. The rise in blood glucose levels is indicated by a food's glycemic index (GI): the faster and higher the blood glucose rise, the higher the GI. The GIs of various foods are shown in Table 1.1.

Sometimes it is an advantage to consume high-GI carbohydrates— for instance, during the first two hours after exercise or towards the end of a long, hard workout when glycogen stores are low. Studies have shown that consuming approximately 1 gram of carbohydrate per kilogram of body weight within the two-hour postexercise period speeds up glycogen refueling and therefore speeds recovery time. In contrast, there are times when it is beneficial to consume lower-GI carbohydrates in a form in which they are absorbed more slowly over a long period (for example, between workouts, or 2 to 4 hours before a workout). This may be achieved either by selecting moderate- and low-GI carbohydrates or by combining high-GI carbohydrates with low-GI carbohydrates, protein, or fat. For example, combine rice (high GI) with beans (low GI); baked potato (high GI) with tuna (protein); or bread (high GI) with cheese (protein and fat).

To enable you to choose the right carbohydrates for the right occasion, refer to Table 1.1.

How Often Should I Eat?

Eating five or six meals or snacks a day at regularly spaced intervals will help to maximize glycogen storage and energy levels, minimize fat storage, stabilize blood glucose and insulin levels, and control blood cholesterol levels. Each time you eat carbohydrate, insulin is produced, which allows glucose, amino acids, and fatty acids to be removed from the bloodstream and taken up by cells. Therefore, eating moderately and frequently causes a relatively steady insulin release, whereas eating most of your food in one or two large meals causes a more rapid insulin release and less effective glycogen storage. There is also a greater chance of some carbohydrate being converted into fat rather than glycogen.

When Should I Eat?

Before a Workout

Eating a snack meal of low- to moderate-GI carbohydrate (for example, pasta with chicken or beans) about 2 to 4 hours before exercise will help prolong a moderate blood glucose rise. Then, eating 25 to 50 grams of high-GI carbohydrate (for example, one or two bananas) just prior to your workout will help increase blood glucose and sustain a higher level for longer in the bloodstream. The optimal timing of this will vary from 5 to 20 minutes before exercise, depending on the individual.

During a Workout

If you are exercising hard for more than 1 hour, consuming 30 to 60 grams of carbohydrate per hour can help delay fatigue and maintain exercise intensity. The amount depends on your body size (the bigger you are, the more carbohydrate energy you expend) and exercise intensity (the harder you exercise, the more carbohydrate energy you expend). This carbohy-

Table 1.1: *Glycemic Index of Various Foods (Glucose = 100)*

High		Moderate		Low	
Grains		**Grains**		**Legumes**	
White bread	69	Whole-meal pasta	42	Butter beans	36
Whole-meal bread	72	White pasta	50	Baked beans	40
Brown rice	80	Oats	49	Green beans	31
		Barley	22	Chickpeas	36
				Lentils	29
				Kidney beans	29
				Soybeans	15
Breakfast cereals		**Breakfast cereals**			
Cornflakes	80	Porridge	54		
Muesli	66	All Bran	51		
Shredded Wheat	67				
Weetabix	75				
Fruit		**Fruit**		**Fruit**	
Raisins	64	Grapes	44	Apples	39
Bananas	62	Oranges	40	Cherries	23
				Plums	25
				Apricots	30
				Grapefruit	26
				Peaches	29
Vegetables		**Vegetables**			
Corn	59	Sweet potato	48		
Parsnips	97	Potato chips	51		
Potato, baked	98	Yam	51		
Carrots	92				
				Dairy products	
				Milk	32
				Yogurt	36
				Ice cream	36
Other		**Other**		**Other**	
Chocolate cookie	59	Oatmeal cookie	54	Fructose	20
Mars Bar	68	Sponge cake	46		
Honey	87				
Sucrose	59				
Glucose	100				
Diluted orange or other fruit juice	66				

drate may be taken in either liquid or solid form. Some people prefer to take a carbohydrate-containing drink, for example an isotonic sports drink or diluted juice, while others prefer to eat carbohydrate in food form, for example bananas and raisins, and to drink water. The choice is yours.

After a Workout

It is most important to start refueling as soon as possible after exercise, as this is when glycogen manufacture is at its most efficient. Studies have shown that eating carbohydrate (1 gram per kilogram of body weight) during the first 2 hours after exercise improves the efficiency of the refueling mechanism by 5 to 7 percent. Choose high-GI carbohydrates during this period, for example, isotonic drinks, bananas, or rice cakes and jam.

How Much Protein?

Active people need more protein per kilogram of body weight than sedentary people in order to compensate for increased protein breakdown during training and to promote new muscle growth and tissue repair. Scientists at the 1991 Lausanne conference on sports nutrition recommended a protein intake of 1.2 to 1.7 g/kg body weight each day. In general, the lower end of the range should cover the needs of most endurance/aerobic athletes, and the upper end of the range is more appropriate for those involved in strength and power sports. For example, if you weigh 60 kg (132 pounds), aim to consume between 72 grams and 102 grams of protein per day. In practice, this should represent 12 to 15 percent of your total energy intake if you are consuming enough calories to meet your needs (i.e., not dieting). Consult Table 1.2 to help you work out your daily intake.

What Are the Best Sources of Protein?

You can get protein from many different foods, and no one source is necessarily better than another. The usefulness of a particular protein is often measured by its biological value (BV), which indicates how closely matched the proportion of amino acids is in relation to the body's requirements. Egg white has a BV of 100, which means that it contains all the essential amino acids that the body requires in closely matched proportions. Therefore, virtually all of the protein provided in the food can be used for making new body proteins.

Other foods with a high BV include milk, cheese, yogurt, meat, fish, poultry, eggs, and soy products.

There are many foods that contain significant amounts of protein but that are short of one or two essential amino acids. These have a low BV and include beans, lentils, peas, bread, cereals, grains, nuts, and seeds. (Soy and a grain called quinoa are the only plant products that contain high-BV protein.) Eating a mixture of low-BV sources during the day is as good as eating proteins with a high BV. In other words, it is not essential to obtain your protein needs purely from animal sources; consuming a variety of both low- and high-BV protein foods is a healthy way to meet your requirements.

Table 1.2: Protein Content of Various Foods

Food	Protein (grams per portion)
Meat/fish/poultry	
Red meat (4 oz.)	32
Chicken (6 oz.)	38
White fish (6 oz.)	30
Oily fish (6 oz.)	30
Sausages (2 med.)	15
Ground beef (4 oz.)	25
Canned tuna (4 oz.)	25
Dairy products and eggs	
Milk (1/2 pint)	10
Cottage cheese (4 oz.)	15
Cheddar cheese (2 oz.)	14
Yogurt (6 oz.)	8
Eggs (2 med.)	14
Legumes and nuts	
Kidney beans (8 oz. boiled)	15
Baked beans (1/2 large tin)	10
Lentils (8 oz. boiled)	15
Nuts (2 oz.)	13
Grains	
Bread (2 slices)	6
Pasta (6 oz. boiled)	5
Rice (6 oz. boiled)	4
Other	
Tofu (4 oz.)	9

Why Do Active Women Need Fat?

It is important to realize that some body fat is absolutely vital. This is called essential fat and includes the fat that forms part of your cell membranes, brain tissue, nerve sheaths, and bone marrow and which surrounds your organs (heart, liver, kidneys), providing insulation, protection, and cushioning against physical damage. In a healthy person, this fat accounts for about 3 percent of body weight. Women have an additional fat requirement called sex-specific fat, which is stored mostly in the breasts and around the hips. This fat is involved in estrogen production and so ensures normal hormone balance and menstrual function. If it becomes too low, hormonal imbalance and menstrual irregularities result. This fat accounts for a further 5 to 9 percent of a woman's body weight.

Fat is also an important energy store, providing 9 calories per gram. It is used during sleep and while sitting, standing, and walking, as well as during aerobic exercise. This fat comes from adipose tissue (fat tissue) distributed all over your body and also from the fat within the muscle cells (particularly important during exercise). One kilogram of adipose tissue could supply enough energy for 15 to 20 hours of exercise. Your fat store is certainly not a redundant depot of unwanted energy!

So, what is a desirable body fat percentage for health? Doctors and physiologists recommend a *minimum* of 5 percent for men and 10 percent for women to cover the most basic functions. In practice, a healthy range for men is between 13 and 18 percent, and for women between 18 and 25 percent. Athletes are likely to be a little lower. One study of elite athletes found that the men had 4 to 10 percent body fat and the women 13 to 18 percent. However, these are not necessarily recommended levels for health.

How Much Fat Is Recommended?

Fat should contribute less than 30 percent of your total energy intake. (Refer to the method earlier in this chapter for calculating percentages of macronutrient intake.) This is in line with the recommendations of the World Health Organization and is aimed at reducing the risk of heart disease and cancer in the general population. In practice, exercisers who are training to lose weight/fat are usually advised to obtain less than 25 percent of their energy from fat. For those who have high energy needs (3,000 calories or more), fat should contribute between 25 and 30 percent of their energy, since it is an energy-dense nutrient.

However, you should not reduce your fat intake to below 15 or 20 percent of energy intake, as this can lead to several nutritional problems. If you do, for example, you are unlikely to consume adequate essential fatty acids (linoleic acid and linolenic acid, found in vegetable oils, seeds, nuts, and oily fish). These fatty acids make up the structure of cell membranes and are needed to produce hormonelike substances called prostaglandins and leukotrienes which help to regulate blood clotting and viscosity, the tone of capillary/artery-wall muscles, the widening and constriction of blood vessels, inflammatory responses, and your immune system.

The fat-soluble vitamins, A, D, E, and K, are found only in fat-containing foods, and some fat is needed to enable your body to absorb and transport them. Although you can get vitamin D from ultraviolet light, vitamin K from dark-green leafy vegetables, and vitamin A from its precursor, beta-carotene, found in brightly colored fruits and vegetables, getting enough vitamin E can be more of a challenge. Vitamin E is found in significant quantities only in vegetable oils, seeds, nuts, and egg yolk. An important antioxidant that protects our cells from harmful free-radical[1] attack, vitamin E is thought to help prevent heart disease and certain cancers and even to retard aging. It may also help to reduce muscle soreness after hard exercise. So, remember that reducing your fat too far may lead to nutritional and health problems.

What Are My Vitamin and Mineral Needs?

Vitamins and minerals play an important role in achieving optimal health and performance. Regular exercise increases the need for many vitamins and minerals, and these can be met from a well-planned, balanced diet that also meets your energy requirements. Although individual needs vary, in the U.S., the Food and Nutrition Board of the National Academy of Sciences, in conjunction with Health Canada, has worked over the last decade to update the Recommended Dietary Allowances, or RDAs. Table 1.3 shows the RDAs for women for most vitamins and minerals. These are the amounts judged to meet the needs of 97 to 98 percent of all individuals in each group.

What About Taking *Extra* Vitamins and Minerals?

There is currently no evidence that vitamin and mineral supplements improve performance if you are already meeting your needs from your diet. However, if your diet is low in a particular nutrient, this is likely to have an adverse effect on your health and performance, and so supplements may have a temporary benefit. Women who are on restricted diets (for example, on weight-loss or vegan diets) and those who have an eating disorder are likely to be lacking in several vitamins or minerals. You should seek professional advice from your physician or a qualified sports nutritionist rather than taking supplements indiscriminately.

Putting the theory into practice is not always easy, especially if you must travel a lot, eat out, or rely on other people to provide your food, and therefore a general multivitamin and mineral supplement may be a wise precaution. There is promising and growing evidence that antioxidant nutrients help to reduce the risks of free-radical damage and therefore may help

Table 1.3: *Dietary Reference Intakes for Women: Recommended Daily Intakes for Individuals*

Nutrient	9–13 years	14–18 years	19–30 years	31–50 years	51–70 years
Thiamine (mg)	0.9	1.0	1.1	1.1	1.1
Riboflavin (mg)	0.9	1.0	1.1	1.1	1.1
Niacin (mg)	12	14	14	14	14
Vitamin B6 (mg)	1.0	1.2	1.3	1.3	1.5
Vitamin B12 (μg)	1.8	2.4	2.4	2.4	2.4†
Folate (μg)	300	400‡	400‡	400‡	400
Vitamin C (mg)	45	65	75	75	75
Vitamin A (μg)	600	700	700	700	700
Calcium (mg)	1,300*	1,300*	1,000*	1,000*	1,200*
Iron (mg)	8	15	18	18	8
Zinc (mg)	8	9	8	8	8
Magnesium (mg)	240	360	310	320	320

(Source: from the Food and Nutrition Board, Institute of Medicine—National Academy of Sciences, 2001)

Note: This table presents Recommended Dietary Allowances (RDAs), except for numbers followed by an asterisk (*), which are Adequate Intakes (AIs). RDAs and AIs may both be used as goals for individual intake. RDAs are set to meet the needs of almost all (97 to 98 percent) individuals in a group. The AI is believed to cover the needs of all individuals in the group, but lack of data or uncertainty in the data prevents being able to specify with confidence the percentage of individuals covered by this intake.

† Because 10 to 30 percent of older people may malabsorb food-bound B12, it is advisable for those older than 50 years to meet their RDA mainly by consuming foods fortified with B12 or a supplement containing B12.

‡ In view of evidence linking folate intake with neural tube defects in the fetus, it is recommended that all women capable of becoming pregnant consume 400 μg from supplements or fortified foods in addition to intake of food folate from a varied diet.

protect against cancer, heart disease, and premature aging. They may also help to alleviate muscle soreness resulting from severe exercise.

Do Women Have Any Special Vitamin or Mineral Requirements?

In general, women tend to have lower intakes of calcium, iron, riboflavin, and folic acid than men. Calcium is important for bone health, and there is evidence that low intakes during childhood and early adulthood may exacerbate other problems common among female exercisers, such as low body fat/weight, overtraining, amenorrhea (absence of periods), psychological stress, and eating disorders. A combination of two or more of these factors increases the risk of stress fractures and osteoporosis in later life. This is discussed in greater detail in Chapter 4. All active women should aim to consume at least the RDA for calcium. Scientists also recommend that women who are amenorrheic should consume 1,200 to 1,500 mg of calcium daily. Good sources of calcium include milk, cheese, yogurt, figs, legumes, oranges, sardines, shellfish, white (fortified) bread and flour, nuts, and green leafy vegetables.

Iron deficiency anemia is more common among female exercisers than male. A large proportion of women have depleted iron stores, which in itself is not a problem but which may easily develop into iron deficiency anemia if the body's iron requirements suddenly increase (for example, during pregnancy). This is usually due to iron loss through menstruation and to generally low iron intake. Many women avoid red meat (which provides one of the richest and most readily absorbed sources of iron) or eat only very small amounts, so they need to make sure that they obtain enough iron from other foods such as legumes, whole-grain cereals, fortified breakfast cereals, and dark-green vegetables. Vitamin C improves iron absorption, so include foods rich in vitamin C (fruit, vegetables, or juices) at the same time. Iron supplements are not routinely recommended for active women, but if you suspect that you may be anemic you should consult your doctor for a blood test and a proper diagnosis. More information about iron deficiency and sports anemia is presented in Chapter 3.

Exercise increases the requirement for riboflavin (vitamin B12), one of the vitamins involved in energy production. Women on low-calorie diets should include plenty of riboflavin-rich foods in their diet, such as milk (this includes low-fat milk), cheese, yogurt, meat, and eggs.

Women generally tend to have low intakes of folic acid (also called folate), one of the B vitamins involved in cell division and red-blood-cell formation. This is particularly important during the first three months of pregnancy, since low intakes may increase the risk of neural-tube defects in the fetus. As a precaution, and as spelled out in Table 1.3 above, the National Academy of Sciences advises that all women capable of becoming pregnant consume 400 µg of folate from supplements or fortified foods. This is discussed in more detail in Chapter 2.

Special Nutritional Considerations for Children and Teenagers

Childhood, puberty, and adolescence are periods of rapid growth. During these times, changes in body size, shape, and composition take place, especially during the pubescent growth spurt (between 9 and 13 years), and these inevitably increase the requirements for energy (calories) and therefore for most nutrients. Children and teenagers involved in sports and exercise are often put under considerable pressure to excel by parents or coaches. They are frequently given well-meaning but misguided advice which can result in various nutrition-related problems such as impaired growth and development, weight problems, eating disorders, and dehydration.

How Do the Nutritional Requirements of Children and Teenagers Differ from Those of Adults?

The nutritional requirements of children and teenagers per pound of body weight are higher than those of adults because kids are growing quickly and gaining lean body weight. Therefore, their energy intake must be sufficient to support their growth rate as well as their activity level. Table 1.4 gives the recommended average energy requirements, but bear in mind that these do not take into account regular exercise or physical training, which may amount to an extra 500 or more calories per day. The exact amount will depend on the type, intensity, frequency, and duration of training. Also, children are generally less efficient in their movements than adults; in other words, they burn more calories per pound of body weight and may use 20 to 30 percent more oxygen per pound of body weight to run at the same speed as adults.

Table 1.4: *Estimated Average Caloric Requirements for Children and Teenagers*

Age	Estimated Average Requirement (calories/day)
7–10 years	1,740
11–14 years	1,845
15–18 years	2,110

(Source: British Department of Health, 1991)

The intake recommendations for carbohydrate (60 percent of caloric intake), fat (20 to 30 percent of caloric intake), and protein (15 percent of caloric intake) are the same for active children and teenagers as they are for adults. In other words, although their *total* energy intake may be different, the optimal *proportions* of carbohydrate, fat, and protein are no different. A word of caution about carbohydrate foods, though: if the child's requirements are high, do not expect her to obtain all her carbohydrate from bulky, high-fiber foods—she may not be able to eat enough. Coaches and parents sometimes forget that children have smaller stomachs, and they apply healthy eating recommendations designed for overweight and sedentary adults to their children with adverse effects. A mixture of bulky, fiber-rich foods (for example, whole-meal bread, whole-meal pasta, and beans) and less bulky, low-fiber foods (for example, white bread, sweetened breakfast cereals, and sweets) may be more appropriate for active children and teenagers.

How Does Children's Body Composition Differ from That of Adults?

The bodies of children and teenagers have a higher water content and a lower bone mineral content, and therefore a lower body density than adults. For this reason, the equations normally used for assessing body fat in adults are not suitable for children—they tend to overestimate fatness by 3 to 6 percent and to underestimate lean body mass. Also, there is a continual fluctuation in kids' fat-free body components. Special equations for estimating body fat from body-density measurements and skinfold-thickness measurements should therefore be used.

Body composition measurements can be used professionally to monitor changes during a training season and to check that normal development is not impaired. It should be stressed that children should not be put on a standard weight-reduction program. A restrictive diet and/or intense exercise program to lose fat can seriously harm a child's physical and psychological development.

Should Active Children and Teenagers Cut Down on Fat?

Young, active exercisers do not necessarily have to cut down on fat. It is recommended that they get 20 to 30 percent of their energy from fats. Remember that some fat in the diet is vital: fats found in vegetable oils, nuts, seeds, and oily fish provide the essential fatty acids which are needed for making prostaglandins (types of hormones) and for the development of nerve and brain tissue. These foods are also good sources of vitamin E, an important antioxidant that helps combat free radicals. Some fat is also needed for absorbing vitamins A, D, E, and K from food.

Fat is also used for energy during rest and exercise. If children eliminate all fatty foods they may not meet their energy requirements.

Perhaps the most important change to encourage in kids is in the *types* of fats eaten. A study carried out at Newcastle University found that about 25 percent of schoolchildren's fat intake came from meat, meat pies, burgers, and sausages, all rich in saturated fats. Children and teenagers should be encouraged to choose lean versions of meat and to include some foods that are rich in unsaturated fats.

Are Children and Teenagers More Likely to Become Dehydrated?

Yes, children have a higher tendency towards heat-related illness than adults. Children do not tolerate extreme temperatures as well as adults because they have a poorer ability to thermoregulate. In other words, their bodies respond differently to exercise: they produce less sweat per sweat gland and so do not perspire as readily, and they produce more heat but are less able to transfer this heat from the muscles to the skin. The smaller the child, the greater this excess heat production.

During exercise, children experience a faster rise in their body's core temperature and so are more easily dehydrated than adults. The problem is that children do not instinctively drink enough to replace their fluid losses and often do not recognize the symptoms of dehydration. Since they also acclimatize more slowly to heat, they need to reduce their training intensity for a while and then to build it up again gradually.

Given that children do not recognize dehydration or voluntarily drink enough, it is important that the drink be highly palatable. Water is not so readily drunk and often quenches the immediate thirst sensation before enough has been drunk to rehydrate the body. Flavored drinks are more appealing. Diluted fruit juice (with a juice-to-water ratio between 1:1 and 1:2) or a commercial sports drink will encourage the child to drink more and also will help her to replace fluids faster (see also Chapter 9, on competition preparation).

Should Children and Teenagers Be Encouraged to Lose Weight?

Embarking on any restrictive diet or on an excessive exercise program with the aim of losing weight can be dangerous during childhood or adolescence. It can harm physical development and lead to long-term psychological problems. Low-calorie or low-fat diets are unlikely to support growth and often result in low intakes of protein, iron, calcium, and vitamins. Unfortunately, many teenage girls are overly concerned about their appearance and weight and restrict their food intake in an attempt to change their body shape. This can often set the stage for disordered eating patterns and eating disorders later on (see Chapter 8, on body image).

If a genuine weight problem exists, or if a child is required to make a weight class for competition, then professional help should be obtained from a qualified sports nutritionist.

The combination of chronic food restriction and high energy demands in youths can lead to:

- glycogen depletion and fatigue
- lowered nutritional status
- reduced immune function

- increased susceptibility to infection and illness
- hormonal disturbances
- menstrual irregularities
- reduced bone density
- eating disorders

Should Children and Teenagers Consume More Calcium?

Calcium is particularly important for the proper development of the skeleton. Between 85 and 90 percent of peak bone mass is achieved by the age of 20, and approximately 45 percent is gained during puberty. The recommended dietary allowance (RDA) for girls 18 and under is 1,300 mg, slightly more than that for adult women, to take into account the increasing bone mass. Results from a 1989 British Department of Health survey of schoolchildren's diets revealed that girls ages 14 and 15 consumed an average of 692 mg of calcium per day; this low intake may result in a lower peak bone mass and a greater risk of osteoporosis. However, many factors affect bone mass and bone mineral density, including diet, exercise, and genetics.

One study has found that children with a higher than average milk (therefore calcium) consumption had a higher calcium retention and bone mineral density than children with a lower intake.

A study carried out in the 1990s at the Royal National Hospital in Bath, England, found a direct link between body weight, bone mineral content, and bone mineral density in children ages 5, 10, and 21 years. Therefore, growth rate appears to be an important factor determining adult bone mass. This is another good reason why children should not embark on diets or restrict their food intake to lose weight.

Do Children and Teenagers Need Extra Iron?

The RDA for iron for girls increases at age 14 from 8 mg to 15 mg. During this growth period, extra iron is needed because of the expansion of blood volume and increased tissue mass associated with growth. The onset of menstruation increases iron loss and therefore increases iron requirements. Many teenage girls are at high risk of iron deficiency anemia due to poor eating habits (for example, dieting, vegetarianism, insufficient iron-rich foods). One study on girls with mild anemia (hemoglobin less than 12 grams per deciliter) showed that they had a lower aerobic capacity than those with normal hemoglobin levels. Good sources of iron include red meat, organ meats, green leafy vegetables, fortified breakfast cereals, and legumes. Vitamin C enhances the absorption of iron. For more information on this topic, refer to Chapter 3, "Iron and Sports Anemia."

Special Nutritional Considerations for the Older Athlete

More and more women are taking up or continuing exercise programs and sports in their later years. Certainly, age is no barrier to exercise and fitness. However, as we get older a number of physiological and functional changes take place, and some of these can have a bearing on nutritional status.

Do Women Go into Functional Decline?

Normally, the aging process is accompanied by a number of physiological changes. These include:

- a reduction in lean mass of up to 20–30 percent, with a selective loss of fast-twitch (type II) muscle fibers

- a reduction in muscle strength

- a reduction in aerobic capacity (up to 30 percent)

- a reduction in growth-hormone production, leading to reduced lean mass

- a reduction in basal metabolic rate (around 10 percent), and therefore a reduction in calorie requirements

- a reduced immune function and increased susceptibility to infection

- a reduction in flexibility (up to 30 percent)

However, none of these changes are inevitable, and they can be prevented—or the risk of them drastically reduced—by regular exercise. Lean body tissue can be maintained through appropriate strength training, and this maintains the basal metabolic rate. Getting older does not mean that your metabolism automatically slows; changes are related to your total body mass and your lean tissue mass. So, most of the functional changes associated with aging are due to a decrease in activity.

Are Older Exercisers More Prone to Dehydration?

Studies have shown that, due to age-related changes in the skin, blood flow to the skin is reduced in older exercisers. Since blood flow to the skin allows heat to be removed by convection from the body core to the skin, sweating ability may arguably be slightly impaired as one ages, with the result that heat is less easily dissipated. Thirst sensation may also be impaired in some people, and this may exacerbate dehydration.

However, older athletes are equally capable of acclimatizing to heat as young athletes. There is a small reduction in thermoregulation, but this is unlikely to impair one's performance, provided one drinks enough fluid (see Chapter 9, on competition preparation).

Do Older Exercisers Need Extra Calcium?

It is important to maintain an adequate calcium intake after peak bone mass has been achieved (between 30 and 40 years), but taking extra calcium from food or supplements will not prevent bone loss (osteoporosis). There is some evidence that the age-related loss of bone mass can be slowed down by regular weight-bearing or strength exercise and/or hormone replacement. However, the value of ingesting calcium over and above the RDA is doubtful.

Do Older Exercisers Need Extra Vitamins?

Antioxidants may help to prevent or delay some of the signs of premature aging. At the moment, this evidence comes from studies on laboratory animals, but research on humans is underway and looks promising.

Antioxidants help to neutralize free radicals. Beta-carotene, vitamin C, and vitamin E are perhaps the most well known and well researched antioxidants, but there are dozens of other natural substances in food (for example, flavenoids and carotenoids) as well as a number of minerals (for example, zinc and selenium) which also have antioxidant properties.

Table 1.5: Dietary Sources of Beta-carotene, Vitamin C, and Vitamin E

Beta-carotene (per 100 g or 3.5 oz.) Suggested optimal intake is 15–25 mg/day†

■ Carrots (boiled)	7.6 mg
■ Red peppers (raw)	3.8 mg
■ Spinach (boiled)	3.8 mg
■ Spring greens (boiled)	2.2 mg
■ Sweet potatoes (boiled)	4.0 mg
■ Mango	1.8 mg
■ Cantaloupe	1.0 mg
■ Dried apricots	0.7 mg

Vitamin C (per 100 g or 3.5 oz.) Suggested optimal intake is 100–150 mg/day†

■ Blackcurrants	200 mg
■ Strawberries	77 mg
■ Oranges	54 mg
■ Tomatoes	17 mg
■ Broccoli (boiled)	44 mg
■ Green peppers (raw)	120 mg
■ Baked potato	14 mg

Vitamin E (per 100 g or 3.5 oz.) Suggested optimal intake is 50–80 mg/day†

■ Sunflower oil	49 mg
■ Safflower oil	40 mg
■ Olive oil	5 mg
■ Sunflower seeds	38 mg
■ Almonds	24 mg
■ Peanuts (plain)	10 mg
■ Peanut butter	5 mg

† In the UK there are no recommended amounts set for any of the antioxidants except vitamin C (40 mg). The U.S., on the other hand, makes recommendations for vitamins C, A (beta-carotene), and E. Several scientists, however, including Professor Anthony Diplock from the University of London at Guys Hospital, believe that the UK- and U.S.-recommended intakes are too low, and Diplock has proposed optimal intakes to give greater protection from disease. For beta-carotene, the optimal level would be 15–25 mg; for vitamin C, 100–150 mg; and for vitamin E, 50–80 mg—all of which are considerably greater than current average intakes.

Hard exercise can deplete the body's antioxidant stores if you don't step up your intake. In a recent study, runners were given either an antioxidant supplement or a placebo pill. After 6 weeks, those who had taken the antioxidant exhibited less free-radical damage than those who took the placebo.

Research suggests that antioxidants may play an important role in protecting muscle fibers from free-radical damage during exercise and in reducing postexercise soreness. At the University of Birmingham, researchers gave volunteers supplements of vitamin C and vitamin E before and after performing 1 hour of step aerobics using the same lead leg. They found that those who had taken the vitamin C supplements experienced less muscle damage, and their recovery was quicker. It was suggested that this was due to vitamin C's antioxidant properties, which helped to protect the muscle-cell membranes.

Which Foods Are Good Sources of Antioxidants?

Fruits and vegetables contain many of the antioxidant nutrients. The World Health Organization recommends five or more portions of fruit and vegetables a day—that's about 400 grams. At the moment, British people on average eat only 250 grams. Nuts, seeds, and their oils are the richest sources of vitamin E. More evidence is accumulating that red wine may help to protect against free-radical damage, probably due to its protective effect on LDL cholesterol from oxidation. Red-wine drinking may help to explain the so-called French paradox: the question of why the French have such a low rate of heart disease despite their high-fat diet and high smoking rate. Red wine contains flavenoids from the red grape skins.

Some scientists say that it is difficult to obtain the appropriate levels of vitamin E and beta-carotene from diet alone, so supplements may be the answer. Others are more cautious in making recommendations and go along with the World Health Organization's emphasis on fruit and vegetable intake.

═Practical Points ═

- Carbohydrate is the most important source of energy for exercise; a low intake can reduce performance and increase fatigue, while an optimal intake can have a significant improvement on training gains, recovery, and performance.

- It is recommended that carbohydrates make up at least 60 percent of one's total energy intake.

- Carbohydrate foods that contain a "package" of other nutrients should form the majority of one's carbohydrate intake, but sugars can also play a valuable role.

- It is important to consider the glycemic index (GI) of the carbohydrate source: high-GI carbohydrates are most beneficial consumed immediately prior to exercise, during exercise lasting more than 1 hour, and within the 2-hour period after exercise.

- An active woman's protein requirements are higher than those of sedentary women. An intake of between 1.2 g and 1.7 g per kg of body weight per day is recommended to cover the needs of most exercisers; this translates into approximately 12–15 percent of total energy (caloric) intake. (To determine body weight in kilograms, divide body weight in pounds by 2.2.)

- Fat should supply between 20 and 30 percent of your total energy intake.

- Very low fat intakes should be avoided. Fat is needed for cell membranes, for protecting the organs, and for ensuring normal hormonal balance; dietary fat is a source of essential fatty acids, fat-soluble vitamins, and energy.

- Vitamin and mineral requirements are generally satisfied by a well-planned and -balanced diet. Higher intakes do not necessarily improve performance or health, although low intakes can have an adverse effect.

- Active women should pay special attention to calcium, iron, riboflavin, and folic acid intakes.

- For optimal performance, aim for 4–5 g of carbohydrate per kilogram of body weight per day if you do less than 1 hour of exercise per day; 5–6 g/kg/day if you exercise 1 hour/day; 6–7 g/kg/day if you exercise 1–2 hours/day; 7–8 g/kg/day if you exercise 2 to 4 hours/day; or 8 to 10 g/kg/day if you exercise more than 4 hours/day.

- For fast refueling and recovery, divide your food intake into five or six moderate-sized meals and snacks per day.

- Have a high-carbohydrate meal 2–4 hours before exercise, followed by a snack containing 25–50 grams of carbohydrate (for example, one or two bananas) just before exercise.

- If you exercise hard for more than 1 hour, consuming an extra 30–60 g/hour of carbohydrate in liquid or solid form will help to delay fatigue (500–1,000 ml of isotonic sports drink or two to three bananas plus water).

- Have a high-carbohydrate snack within 2 hours after exercise (for example, a banana sandwich).

- Consume a variety of protein sources, including foods with a high biological value (milk, poultry, eggs) and foods with a low biological value (legumes, grains).

- Keep your fat intake below 30 percent of your total energy intake, but do not reduce it too severely. Include the equivalent of 1–2 tablespoonfuls of vegetable oil, nuts, or seeds per day in order to obtain the essential fatty acids and allow your body to absorb fat-soluble vitamins such as vitamin E.

- Aim to obtain all of your vitamins and minerals from nutrient-rich foods. Consider a general multivitamin and mineral supplement if you are on a weight-reducing diet, travel, or eat out a lot. Antioxidant supplements may have health benefits and reduce the risk of damage from free radicals.

- Do not take individual vitamin or mineral supplements indiscriminately without the advice of a sports nutritionist.

Further Reading

A. Bean, *The Complete Guide to Sports Nutrition* (A & C Black, 1993).

F. Brouns, *Nutritional Needs of Athletes* (Wiley, 1994).

"Foods, Nutrition and Sports Performance" (*Journal of Sports Sciences*, vol. 9, special issue, 1991).

International Journal of Sports Nutrition (Human Kinetics Publishers, Inc.).

N. Clark, *Nancy Clark's Sports Nutrition Guidebook* (Leisure Press, 1989).

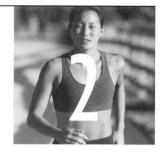

Nutrition During Pregnancy

Anita Bean, B.Sc.

It is generally accepted that a nutritious, balanced diet during pregnancy plays a vital role in both the development of the baby and in the mother's continued good health. There is also increasing evidence that dietary intake during pregnancy has long-term consequences for the child, affecting in particular the risk of heart disease, stroke, diabetes, and bronchitis in later life (this concept is known as "early programming").

Many exercising women worry that the physical and psychological demands of regular training may affect their chances of conception and of a successful pregnancy. They may ask themselves, "Can a lower than average body weight and level of body fat have an adverse effect on the outcome of my pregnancy?" or "Should I eat for two during this time, or try to restrict my weight gain to avoid unnecessary fat stores?"

This chapter helps to answer these and other questions by presenting the latest recommendations on pregnancy, nutrition, and exercise and by offering practical advice on overcoming the dietary problems that are commonly encountered during this life stage. The chapter will help you to understand and meet your nutritional needs so that both you and your baby stand the best possible chance of good health—both now and in the future.

Can I Get Pregnant If I Have a Low Body-Fat Level?

Low body fat and low body weight are often associated with reduced sex-hormone levels and reduced fertility. The threshold below which ovulation and menstruation stop (amenorrhea) is usually between 15 and 20 percent body fat or a body mass index (BMI) of less than 20. (See Chapter 6 for an

Table 2.1: *Body Composition Changes During Pregnancy*

Body component	Increase in weight (kg x 2.2 = lbs.)
Baby	3.4 kg
Placenta	0.65 kg
Amniotic fluid	0.8 kg
Uterus	0.97 kg
Breasts	0.41 kg
Blood	1.25 kg
Extracellular fluid	1.68 kg
Fat	3.35 kg
Total	**12.5 kg**

explanation of how to calculate your BMI.) In order to become pregnant, a certain ratio of body fat to lean body mass is needed. Body fat is important for fertility because it is involved in the production of sex hormones, which are responsible for ovulation. What's more, studies have shown that women with very low body fat tend to produce less potent forms of estrogen.

If you have irregular or absent periods, gaining a little weight and fat will increase your fertility and therefore your chances of successful conception. In practice, a reduction in training intensity and a small increase in food intake is sufficient to bring back normal menstrual cycles.

Your weight and body-fat level before pregnancy are both important for your baby's development and pregnancy outcome. Studies have shown that a low prepregnancy weight increases the risk of a baby with low birth weight.

So make sure that your weight and body fat are within a healthy range before you plan to get pregnant, as this will help to bring about conception and to increase the likelihood of having a baby of optimal weight.

How Much Weight Should I Gain?

On average, most women gain around 12.5 kg (28 lbs.) during a full-term pregnancy of 40 weeks, although anywhere between 11.5 and 16 kg (25–35 lbs.) is considered healthy. About one-quarter of this (3–4 kg/6–9 lbs.) will be the weight of your baby; about half (6 kg/13 lbs.) will be pregnancy-related tissues (placenta, amniotic fluid, uterus, breast tissue, and extra blood); and about one-quarter (3–4 kg/6–9 lbs.) will be laid down as a fat store.

This fat is deposited mainly subcutaneously—that is, just under the skin—in the upper thighs, hips, and abdomen under the influence of the

Table 2.2: *Guidelines for Weight Gain During Pregnancy*

Status at start of pregnancy	Optimal weight gain (in lbs.)	Optimal weight gain (in kg)
Underweight (BMI < 19.8)	28–40 lbs.	12.5–18 kg
Normal weight (BMI 19.8–26)	25–35 lbs.	11.5–16 kg
Overweight (BMI 26–29)	15–25 lbs.	7–11.5 kg
Obese (BMI > 30)	13 lbs. (minimum)	6 kg (minimum)

(Source: U.S. National Academy of Sciences, 1990)

hormone progesterone. Most fat deposition occurs in midpregnancy. This is because it acts as a buffer of stored energy for late pregnancy and breast-feeding, when the energy demands of the baby are highest.

Interestingly, fat mobilization starts in the latter stages of pregnancy and continues for a short while after the birth, as levels of the hormone lactogen rise. In other words, various pregnancy hormones encourage your body to lay down fat midterm and then to mobilize it late- and post-term.

The amount of fat stored during pregnancy varies enormously from woman to woman. In practice, some women gain far more than 3–4 kg of fat—up to 20 kg in extreme cases! In 1990 the Institute of Medicine of the U.S. National Academy of Sciences issued guidelines for optimum weight gain. They suggested that the amount of weight gained depends on how heavy a woman is at the start of pregnancy. If you are overweight, you should aim to gain a little less than the normal recommendation. If you are underweight, you should aim to "catch up" by gaining more than 28 pounds. This greatly improves your chances of having an easy pregnancy.

What Are the Dangers of Putting On Too Much Weight?

Obviously, it is important to avoid putting on too much fat while pregnant. Being overweight and gaining too much weight in pregnancy increase the risk of gestational diabetes, a mild form of diabetes. This is usually only a temporary condition but may occasionally turn out to be a more serious long-term problem. There is also the danger of developing high blood pressure or preeclampsia, which is associated with premature delivery. Very overweight women are more likely to have extra-large babies, who may need forceps or cesarean delivery. So follow the guidelines given in Table 2.2.

What Dangers Are Associated with Being Underweight in Pregnancy?

Being underweight (BMI < 20) or restricting your weight gain if you are not overweight will affect your developing baby. Studies show that a low pregnancy weight gain may seriously retard your baby's growth in the womb and that this can have adverse consequences on later growth (possibly also on neurobehavioral development). The baby is more likely to be underweight when born and shorter in length than normal. Head circumference is also likely to be smaller.

The important message is this: if you are underweight, make sure you put on a minimum of 28 pounds. If you are normal weight, do not overly restrict your weight gain: aim for around 28 pounds. If you are overweight, you should aim for a slightly smaller weight gain, but speak to your doctor or dietitian first.

How Many Calories Should I Eat?

During early pregnancy, the extra amount of food energy required is very small indeed. So, contrary to popular belief, you don't need to eat extra calories at this time. Only during the last 3 months is there a substantial increase in energy needs as the baby grows larger and additional pregnancy-related tissues are laid down. The British Department of Health recommends an extra 200 calories a day at this time. Again, this is not a hard and fast rule as it depends on your weight at the start of pregnancy. Overweight women may need fewer calories than this; underweight women may need more.

Will My Metabolism Change?

It is a common misconception that your metabolic rate drops when you are pregnant. Many women attribute their excess weight (fat) gain to a reduction in their metabolic rate, but this has been shown to be completely untrue.

Researchers at the Dunn Clinical Nutrition Center in Cambridge, England, monitored the metabolic rates of British and Gambian women before and during their pregnancy. Interestingly, they found that the metabolic rate of British women who were slightly plump actually *increased* while they were pregnant! The metabolism of very thin British and Gambian women slowed during pregnancy, presumably due to a need for energy conservation. In other words, the body is remarkably adaptive to a wide range of calorie intakes.

Carbohydrate, fat, and protein metabolism changes during pregnancy due to alterations in hormone levels. Your body's main priority is to help ensure a steady supply of glucose for the baby, so your body adapts to make better use of fats for fuel. Hormonal changes also ensure that your lean tissue is conserved and not broken down for energy unless it proves absolutely necessary.

Doesn't Pregnancy Give You a Weight Problem for Life?

It is quite normal and necessary to gain some extra fat during pregnancy. This is in preparation for breastfeeding and is also nature's safety precaution in case of famine during later pregnancy. Fat gain should amount to 3–4 kg on average, and most (if not all) will be quickly utilized for milk production when you start breastfeeding.

However, there is no reason why pregnancy should give you a long-term weight problem. Studies show that women who gain a lot of excess weight during pregnancy were already overweight or were battling with a weight problem before they became pregnant. Another theory is that before they marry or become pregnant many women suppress their weight by dieting to please the opposite sex. Once they are pregnant and see their body expanding, they give up the dieting battle and use pregnancy as the perfect excuse to overindulge. Hence, the excess weight gain.

Any excess fat gained during pregnancy over and above the normal 3–4 kg can be safely and gradually lost through a combination of a healthy low-fat diet and regular exercise once breastfeeding has ceased (see Chapter 7). It is not recommended to restrict calorie intake during breastfeeding because you risk not obtaining sufficient amounts of key nutrients (e.g., calcium, essential fatty acids) needed for breast-milk production.

Is It Dangerous to Restrict My Food Intake During Pregnancy?

Restricting your food intake can lead to all sorts of problems unless you receive proper professional advice from a nutritionist. It is often difficult for lean athletes to accept increases in their body weight and fat. You may feel tempted to restrict your fat gain by restricting your food intake, but doing so may result in a number of potentially serious problems.

First, you can affect the growth and development of your baby. In general, the lower your calorie intake, the lower the weight of your baby For example, in one study carried out on women living in Hackney, London, low-birthweight babies were more common in those women who had the lowest daily calorie intake (1,600 calories).

Second, if you skip a meal or leave a long gap between meals, your blood-sugar levels will fall. This can have harmful consequences on your developing baby, who relies on a steady supply of blood sugar from your shared bloodstream. Remember, your baby has no energy stores and is therefore totally reliant on a constant supply of fuel and nutrients from you.

Third, there is a danger that you may not get enough nutrients to sustain your own body's stores *and* to feed your baby. Generally, your baby will take what he or she needs from your body, but if your stores run out then he or she may suffer too. The end result could be depleted iron and calcium stores for you and a greater danger of early osteoporosis, unless you keep up your intake of key nutrients such as iron and calcium.

Do I Need Extra Fat in My Diet During Pregnancy?

Certain types of dietary fats are especially important in pregnancy, so you will have to make sure that you include these regularly in your diet. The two essential fatty acids (linoleic acid and linolenic acid) cannot be made in the body. They are converted to arachidonic acid and docosahexanoic acid respectively, which are essential for brain and central nervous system development. They are also needed for cell development and healthy sperm (make sure your partner includes them in his diet). A deficiency of these essential fatty acids may therefore affect your baby's brain development.

Athletes who follow a very low fat diet *must* ensure that they include essential fatty acids in their diet, and this is particularly vital prior to conception and during pregnancy. This may mean slightly increasing the amount of fat you normally eat. Good sources of essential fatty acids include vegetable oils (sunflower, rapeseed), oily fish (sardines, mackerel, salmon), nuts, and seeds. The equivalent of a tablespoon of oil or 25 g (1 ounce) of nuts or seeds a day will give you enough essential fatty acids. Experts also recommend oily fish at least once a week.

Do I Need Extra Vitamins?

During pregnancy there is an increased need for most vitamins and minerals, especially during the last 3 months. Most of the baby's needs are met by your existing stores of minerals and fat-soluble vitamins; nevertheless, most American obstetricians recommend a prenatal vitamin/mineral supplement. Ask your doctor or dietitian for advice.

Table 2.3 shows the RDAs for certain nutrients during pregnancy. Compare these amounts to the RDAs for the same nutrients as shown in Table 1.3 (Chapter 1) for nonpregnant women.

Should I Take Folic Acid Supplements?

The British Department of Health and the National Academy of Sciences (U.S.) both advise that any woman planning a pregnancy should take a supplement of 400 micrograms (0.4 mg) of folic acid per day. This is because a folate deficiency has been linked with a greater risk of neutral tube defects (NTD), such as spina bifida, in newborn babies. Studies have shown that high intakes of this B vitamin (from supplements) taken prior to conception and during early pregnancy can reduce the risk. Although women who have already had an affected baby are at greater risk, the recommendation to increase folate intake applies to all women, because 95 percent of pregnancies affected by an NTD are a first occurrence.

The average adult's daily intake of folic acid is only about 130 micrograms. You can increase your intake by eating more folic acid–rich foods, eating foods fortified with folic acid (some breakfast cereals and bread), or taking folic acid supplements. Fruits, vegetables, and yeast extract are the best food sources of folic acid and offer a range of other nutrients too. Refer to Table 2.4 for more information.

Do I Need Extra Minerals?

The RDAs for most minerals, most significantly iron, increase during pregnancy. This is one more reason why doctors in the United States recommend prenatal supplementation.

Table 2.3: *Dietary Reference Intakes for Pregnant Women: Recommended Daily Intakes*

Nutrient	Up to 18 years	19–30 years	31–50 years
Thiamine (mg)	1.4	1.4	1.4
Riboflavin (mg)	1.4	1.4	1.4
Niacin (mg)	18	18	18
Vitamin B6 (mg)	1.9	1.9	1.9
Vitamin B12 (μg)	2.6	2.6	2.6
Folate (μg)	600†	600†	600†
Vitamin C (mg)	80	85	85
Vitamin A (μg)	750	770	770
Calcium (mg)	1,300n	1,000n	1,000*
Iron (mg)	27	27	27
Zinc (mg)	13	11	11
Magnesium (mg)	400	350	360

(Source: from the Food and Nutrition Board, Institute of Medicine—National Academy of Sciences, 2001)

Note: This table presents Recommended Dietary Allowances (RDAs), except for numbers followed by an asterisk (*), which are Adequate Intakes (AIs). RDAs and AIs may both be used as goals for individual intake. RDAs are set to meet the needs of almost all (97 to 98 percent) individuals in a group. The AI is believed to cover the needs of all individuals in the group, but lack of data or uncertainty in the data prevents being able to specify with confidence the percentage of individuals covered by this intake.

† It is assumed that women will continue consuming 400 μg from supplements or fortified food until their pregnancy is confirmed and they enter prenatal care, which ordinarily occurs after the end of the periconceptional period—the critical time for formation of the neural tube.

Calcium

Calcium is needed for bone and teeth development, and evidence exists that it may also be important in regulating blood pressure during pregnancy. Calcium requirements increase during pregnancy, particularly in the last 10 weeks, when the baby's bones are growing fast. However, there is no recommendation to increase your dietary intake, as your baby's increased needs are met from your existing calcium stores (bones) and also by increasing calcium absorption from food.

Iron

Iron is needed for the manufacture of hemoglobin in red blood cells. More red blood cells are made during pregnancy to help carry oxygen to the baby. About one-third of your iron stores are used for this purpose, so it is important that you get enough iron in your diet to prevent anemia. The absorption of iron from food increases naturally during pregnancy from about 7 to 10 percent upward to 30 to 40 percent towards the end in order to meet your increased needs.

The RDA for iron during pregnancy increases dramatically: from 15 or 18 mg per day (depending on the mother's age) to 27 mg per day. And since many exercisers tend to have low iron stores (although they are not anemic), they may be at risk of iron-deficiency anemia during or after pregnancy. Iron supplements may therefore be advisable; you should check with your doctor. Refer to Table 2.5 for more information.

Zinc

Zinc is involved in cell division and so is essential for your baby's growth. As with iron, some of the additional zinc needed during pregnancy comes from your body's stores and through increased intestinal absorption. Nevertheless, zinc is another mineral whose RDA increases during pregnancy. Zinc is also needed for healthy sperm, so make sure your partner has a plentiful supply if you are planning a pregnancy.

If you have been advised to take iron supplements, you may also need to take zinc supplements or a multivitamin supplement, since a high iron intake can reduce zinc absorption. Consult a sports nutritionist if in doubt.

Table 2.4: *The Folic Acid Content of Various Foods*

Food	Portion size	Folic acid (µg/portion)
Broccoli	100 g	64
Baked potato	200 g	88
Beets	100 g	110
Brussels sprouts	100 g	110
Cabbage	100 g	29
Mushrooms (raw)	50 g	22
Spinach	100 g	90
Banana	One	15
Oranges	One	50
Bran Flakes (fortified)	40 g	100
Cornflakes (fortified)	40 g	100
Yeast extract	4 g	40
Chickpeas (boiled)	150 g	81

Table 2.5: *The Iron Content of Various Foods*

Food	Portion size	Iron (mg/portion)
Beef (average cut)	100 g	2.8
Chicken (meat only)	150 g	1.2
Sardines	50 g	2.3
Lentils (cooked)	120 g	4.0
Baked beans	200 g	2.8
Eggs	2	1.6
Weetabix	2	3.0
Broccoli	100 g	1.0
Spinach	100 g	1.7
Whole-meal bread	2 slices	1.3

What About Food Cravings?

Changes in taste and appetite are common during pregnancy, though whether there is a true physiological basis to this remains open to debate. Many women develop an increased appetite and experience a ravenous desire (craving) for certain foods. If your diet is otherwise well balanced, then this is unlikely to be a problem, especially if your craving is for a fairly healthy food. If you must give in to less healthy cravings, do so only in moderation and make sure that you are still getting enough nutrients from other foods. A good idea is to try healthier options of less nourishing cravings, (e.g., a scone instead of a piece of cake).

Many women wish to eliminate certain fatty and fried foods, alcohol, meat, coffee, and spicy foods during the first few months of their pregnancy. Again, this is not a problem provided the rest of your diet is nutritious and you drink plenty of other fluids, such as herb/fruit teas, water, and diluted fruit juice instead of coffee and tea.

What About Morning Sickness?

More than half of all pregnant women suffer from morning sickness, nausea, or heartburn. These symptoms are thought to be due to dramatic increases in certain hormones, such as human chorionic growth hormone (HCG), produced by the placenta.

Don't worry about your baby, who will draw on your nutrient stores and be well protected against deficiencies. Try to eat small, high-carbohydrate

Table 2.6: *Food Sources of Some Vitamins and Minerals*

Calcium	Low-fat milk, yogurt, cheese, dark-green vegetables, beans, lentils, almonds, sardines, prawns, figs
Iron	Red meat, liver, whole-meal bread, whole-grain or fortified breakfast cereals, dark-green vegetables, beans, lentils
Zinc	Red meat, whole-grain bread and cereals, nuts, seeds, eggs
Folic acid	Green leafy vegetables, liver, whole-grain cereals, eggs, beans, lentils, bananas
Vitamin D	Oily fish, eggs, margarine, fortified breakfast cereals
B vitamins	Whole-grain cereals, legumes, nuts, meat, milk, cheese
Vitamin C	Strawberries, raspberries, black currants, oranges, green vegetables, peppers, orange juice, tomatoes

snacks at regular intervals to ease nausea: a roll and a banana, breakfast cereal, dried fruit, yogurt, or rice cakes with fruit spread. To reduce morning sickness, try crystallized ginger, ginger cookies, plain crackers, or toast. And if you crave strange food combinations, e.g., pickles and ice cream, go ahead. It's better to eat something than nothing at all. Milk-based drinks can alleviate heartburn. Make your own milkshake from low-fat milk, fruit, and yogurt, or use a commercial mix and add milk. Drink plenty of fluids, too.

Should I Avoid Caffeine?

There is no convincing evidence that caffeine in moderation has any adverse effect on pregnancy. Some early studies suggested that high intakes reduced fertility and birth weight and increased the risk of birth defects. However, these have not been proved, and more recent, more comprehensive studies have found no ill effects at all.

During pregnancy your body metabolizes caffeine more slowly, especially during the last 3 months. Caffeine can pass freely from your bloodstream across the placenta into your baby's blood, but there is no evidence of any harm caused by moderate intake. In any case, many pregnant women find that they develop an aversion to coffee and tea; the physiological reason for this is not known.

So, if you like drinking coffee and tea, there is no reason why you should not continue to take in moderate amounts—the equivalent of 4 to 5 cups a day will not do any harm.

Table 2.7: *Sample Daily Eating Plan for a Pregnant Woman*

(Suitable for vegetarians and meat eaters)

Breakfast:	50 g (2 oz.) Bran Flakes, one chopped banana, and 300 ml low-fat milk *or* two to three slices of whole-grain toast with a health fruit spread
Snack:	One piece of fruit; one yogurt or low-fat milk drink
Lunch:	Large baked potato with 100 g (4 oz.) of tuna *or* baked beans with whole-grain toast Side salad with 1 tbsp. dressing Low-fat cottage cheese and fresh fruit
Snack:	Bagel or fruit scone Diluted fruit juice
Dinner:	200 g (8 oz.) cooked pasta with tomato sauce or lean-meat sauce *or* pasta with lentil/vegetable sauce Large portion of vegetables or salad Rice pudding with fruit
Energy:	2,200 calories; 60 percent from carbohydrate; 20 percent from protein; 20 percent from fat

Can I Drink Alcohol?

The occasional drink certainly won't harm you or your baby, but heavy drinking (more than 30 units a week) can lead to stunted growth and retarded mental development—a condition sometimes called fetal alcohol syndrome. Alcohol can pass from your bloodstream across the placenta into your baby's blood, so high levels can affect his or her development.

According to the Royal College of Physicians, it is safest to avoid alcohol altogether, especially during the first 3 months. After that, limit yourself to 1 or 2 units once or twice a week. One unit is equivalent to half a pint of beer, 1 glass of wine, or 1 ounce of spirits.

Is Vitamin A Harmful in Pregnancy?

Vitamin A itself is not harmful; indeed, it is essential for a healthy pregnancy, as it is needed for proper cell division and development. The reason it hit the headlines in the 1990s is because of a few cases reported in the U.S. in which megadose supplements of vitamin A (more than 8,000–10,000 μg per day) led to birth abnormalities. However, these doses were more than ten times the daily requirement (700 μg/day).

As a safety precaution, the British Department of Health advises pregnant women to avoid vitamin A supplements and fish-liver-oil capsules (unless advised by a doctor). It also recommends avoiding liver (and products made from it, such as liver pâté and liver sausage), because these foods sometimes contain very high concentrations of vitamin A. Women should discuss this matter with their obstetrician.

There is no risk from other vitamin A sources, such as milk, cheese, eggs, and carrots, because they contain much smaller concentrations. Only one case of vitamin A toxicity has been recorded in a pregnant woman who ate too much liver. So, in reality, the risk of overdosing on vitamin A is very small indeed!

Am I or Is My Baby at Risk of Listeriosis?

Listeriosis is an illness caused by the listeria bacteria, which contaminate certain foods. It is quite rare and produces flu-like symptoms. It is of concern to pregnant women because it can cause miscarriage, stillbirth, or severe illness in the newborn baby.

Unlike most other bacteria, listeria can multiply at the low temperatures found in refrigerators. It can be a problem with certain cheeses contaminated after manufacture, because they are kept for fairly long periods at low temperatures, thus giving the bacteria a chance to multiply. The British Department of Health advises that pregnant women:

- avoid mold-ripened soft cheeses such as camembert and brie, and also blue-veined cheeses such as blue Stilton (hard cheeses, cottage cheese, and processed cheese are fine)
- reheat "cooked-chilled" foods (for example, ready-made meals) and ready-to-eat poultry until they are piping hot
- avoid pâté and undercooked poultry or meat products
- wash salads, vegetables, and fruit thoroughly
- check the "use by" dates on chilled food
- store cooked and raw foods separately in the fridge

Again, discuss this matter with your obstetrician.

Am I at Risk of Salmonella Poisoning?

Pregnant women are more prone to salmonella poisoning. This won't harm your baby, but it can cause you sickness and diarrhea. Reduce the risks by:

- avoiding raw or lightly cooked eggs and egg-based products (for example, mayonnaise, mousse, uncooked cheesecake)

- make sure eggs are cooked until both the white and yolk are solid

- avoid undercooked chicken

- avoid cross-contamination of uncooked chicken and other foods—keep work surfaces clean and store raw and cooked foods separately in the fridge

- reheat cooked chicken until it is piping hot

Should I Stop Exercising When I'm Pregnant?

There is no reason to stop exercising during pregnancy if you are accustomed to regular training. You can certainly continue to train provided you feel well and are not excessively tired or nauseous, although you may have to make a few modifications to your usual program. Indeed, exercise during pregnancy brings many physiological and psychological benefits. It is not advisable, however, for very unfit women or those who have not previously exercised regularly to embark on an intensive program.

The important difference is that you should now aim to *maintain* rather than *improve* your fitness. In practice, this means reducing your training intensity and volume to a level lower than before. This will not result in a decrease in fitness, because your body is naturally undergoing a training effect during pregnancy. Large increases in estrogen output encourage the development of bone strength and lean tissue mass, including skeletal muscle. The heart muscle becomes stronger, increasing stroke and blood volume. Raised levels of progesterone relax the smooth muscles, including those surrounding the blood vessels, allowing them to accommodate this increased blood volume. All of these changes mimic those resulting from regular physical training.

As pregnancy progresses, gradually reduce your training intensity and volume. Many conditioned women find they can continue exercising until the thirtieth week or longer. There is no recommended cut-off date before the birth, but you should listen carefully to your body, observe the precautions detailed in this chapter, and stop exercising if you notice any of the symptoms listed in Table 2.8 or if the first stage of labor commences.

What Are the Benefits of Regular Exercise During Pregnancy?

Regular exercise maintains good stamina, boosting your ability to deal with the physical demands of pregnancy. Your posture will improve, reducing posture-related problems such as backache, joint prob-

Table 2.8: Reasons to Stop Exercising During Pregnancy

If you experience any of the following symptoms, stop exercising and consult your doctor or midwife:	
■ vaginal bleeding	■ shortness of breath
■ very rapid heartbeat	■ uterine contractions
■ dizziness or faintness	■ back pain
■ pelvic pain	■ abdominal pain
■ nausea	■ excessive fatigue

lems, and lordosis (excessive arching of the lower back). Common pregnancy ailments such as tiredness, nausea, constipation, varicose veins, cramps, and water retention will be alleviated, and the likelihood of excessive fat gain lessened. You will also be paving the way for an easier labor.

Regular exercise brings many psychological benefits, such as reduced stress and anxiety, enhanced feelings of well-being, and improved self-esteem and body image.

There is evidence that exercise in early pregnancy stimulates placental growth and that continued exercise throughout the term may improve placental function by about 30 percent, thereby enhancing placental blood flow to the developing fetus.

Are There Any Special Precautions I Should Take When Exercising?

You should avoid any activity that places excessive pressure or stress upon your joints. Avoid overextending any joint or any activity that causes excessive movement around your joints, as the ligaments (which support the joints) become softer and more lax owing to the effects of the hormone relaxin. The joints most at risk are the pelvic joints and the sacroiliac (lower back) joint, particularly in the second and third trimesters of pregnancy.

For this reason, it is best to avoid prolonged high-impact activities such as running (and any sports which include running), jumping, plyometrics, and high-impact aerobics. You should also avoid using very heavy weights when weight training and pay extra attention to correct technique. To minimize the stress on your joints, it is advisable to modify your program to include low-impact activities such as swimming, walking, low-impact aerobics, light to moderate weight training, light circuit training, water aerobics, and any sport that doesn't involve much running or jumping.

Avoid repetitive stress to your joints and muscles by varying the muscle groups used within a single training session (e.g., by combining lower-body and upper-body exercises) and also by varying the types of activities in your program, i.e., cross-training.

Good technique is even more important during pregnancy to ensure good joint alignment (e.g., hips, knees, ankles), and to avoid unbalanced loads (e.g., during resistance training).

It is important both for your body and your developing baby to ensure that your core body temperature does not exceed 38°C (100°F). Overheating, or hyperthermia, may, in theory, harm the development of your baby and result in fetal growth retardation. To avoid thermal stress, the American College of Obstetricians and Gynecologists recommends that you should limit the duration of strenuous activity to 15 minutes and make sure your heart rate does not exceed 140 beats per minute for an extended period of time. Other sensible precautions include:

- exercising at a low or submaximal level (less than 65 percent of VO_2 max, or maximum aerobic capacity—the maximum volume of oxygen you can consume during physical activity);

- exercising within your maximum exercise intensity based on heart rate (220 minus your age is your maximum heart rate; the training range for aerobic conditioning is between 65 and 85 percent of this maximum);

- ensuring your surroundings are well ventilated and not too warm;

- keeping well hydrated by drinking plenty of fluids;

- and allowing sufficient cool-down time after training.

The risk of thermal stress is smaller for well-conditioned women as they are better able to thermoregulate than those new to exercise.

Think consciously about reducing your training intensity. During pregnancy it is easy to underestimate your exertion due to increased levels of beta-endorphins ("painkiller" hormones produced by the brain), which decrease your perceived rate of exertion.

Should I Avoid Any Particular Exercises?

The American College of Obstetricians and Gynecologists recommends avoiding any exercises performed in the *supine* (lying down) position after the fourth month of pregnancy. This is because of the increased weight of the uterus pressing down on the *vena cava* (the main vein that returns blood to the heart), which can cause a drop in blood pressure, dizziness, and faintness.

For most women, after about the twentieth week of pregnancy the *abdominus recti* separates longitudinally to accommodate the size of the baby. Once this has occurred, you should avoid intensive abdominal exercises, as these cause uneven pressure on the recti, resulting in a "dome" along the *linea alba* (central connective tissue). Sit-ups or crunches should therefore be avoided once the abdomen can no longer be kept flat in the supine position. A recommended alternative abdominal exercise is trunk curls, which are performed on all fours.

Avoid any *hyperextension* (arching) of the back, as this will over-stretch the softened ligaments of the *sacroiliac joint*, resulting in back pain and lordosis. The American College of Obstetricians and Gynecologists also advises against increased intra-abdominal pressure or straining (e.g., when lifting heavy weights or performing resistance exercises), as this can raise blood pressure and restrict blood supply to the fetus. Avoid *isometric* (static or held) exercises (e.g., holding arms overhead for a long period), as these can also increase blood pressure.

What About the Pelvic Floor Muscles?

The pelvic floor muscles hang like a taut hammock between the pubic bone at the front and the coccyx at the back. These support the abdominal contents (i.e., uterus, bladder, intestines, etc.). During pregnancy and labor they come under extra stress, so it is important to help strengthen them by including pelvic floor exercises (Kegel exercises) in your daily routine. This will help prevent some of the common pregnancy discomforts such as hemorrhoids, constipation, and urinary incontinence, and will also prepare the way for an easier childbirth.

Is There Any Other Advice to Follow?

Wear a good supportive bra and correct footwear during exercise to help avoid back and joint problems.

Pay special attention to your posture at all times as this will help minimize strain on your lower back caused by the weight of your uterus pulling down. When standing, lengthen the spine, and keep the abdominals taut, shoulders down, and chest lifted. Your knees should be relaxed. When sitting, keep your spine upright and supported in the region of your lower back, and keep the back of your thighs in contact with the seat. Do not slouch forward.

Learn to listen to your body. Do not exercise if you feel unduly tired, nauseous, or faint. Do not push yourself too hard, and stop if you feel uncomfortable, notice any spotting, or experience any pain, particularly in the pelvic region.

═Practical Points ═

- Low body fat and weight are usually associated with reduced sex-hormone levels and reduced fertility. Chances of conception decrease below a threshold of 15–20 percent body fat or a body mass index (BMI) of 20.

- If you are planning to become pregnant and have irregular or absent periods, you may have to reduce your training intensity and/or increase your body fat a little. This will improve your chances of conception and help ensure an optimal birth weight for your baby.

- A low prepregnancy weight may increase the risk of having a low-birthweight baby.

- The average weight gain during pregnancy is 11.5–16 kg (25–35 pounds); underweight women should aim to gain slightly more;

overweight women should aim to gain slightly less.

- Being underweight (BMI < 20) or intentionally restricting your weight gain in pregnancy can restrict the growth and development of your baby and have adverse long-term consequences.

- Extra calories are not required until the last 3 months of pregnancy, when an additional 200 calories per day are recommended.

- Weight problems post-pregnancy are not inevitable; there is no evidence that pregnancy causes a decreased metabolic rate or excessive fat deposition.

- Your diet should contain enough essential fatty acids to support the growth and development of your baby's brain and central nervous system.

- Do not attempt to restrict your food intake or go on a diet during pregnancy. This may mean your baby will be born shorter and lighter than normal.

- There is an increased need for most vitamins and minerals, but most of these are met by the baby's drawing on your existing stores and through increased intestinal absorption. The most important ones include calcium, iron, zinc, folic acid, vitamin C, vitamin D, and the B vitamins.

- You may continue a regular training program throughout pregnancy— provided you feel well—gradually reducing the training intensity and volume as pregnancy progresses.

- Concentrate on low-impact activities such as swimming, walking, low-impact aerobics, moderate to light weight training, and light circuit training, and avoid prolonged high-impact activities (e.g., running, jumping). Vary the activities in your routine.

- Aim to maintain rather than increase your fitness.

- Because the ligaments are more lax during pregnancy, avoid any activity that places excessive pressure, stress, or movement on any joint. Avoid repetitive stress to your joints, and pay extra attention to correct technique.

- Make sure you avoid any hyperextension of the lower back, and pay strict attention to posture at all times.

- It is recommended that pregnant women avoid any supine exercises, particularly abdominal exercises performed in the supine position, after the twentieth week.

- Avoid thermal stress by using low- or submaximal-intensity activities, limiting strenuous activity to 15 minutes duration, and ensuring your heart rate does not often exceed 140 beats per minute.

- Also avoid thermal stress by ensuring that your body temperature does not exceed 38°C (100°F). Drink plenty of fluids before, during, and after exercise, monitor your heart beat, exercise in well-ventilated surroundings, and allow extra time for cooling down.

- Include plenty of folate-rich foods (fruit and vegetables) in your diet and take a supplement containing 400 μg of folic acid until the twelfth week of pregnancy.

- Include the equivalent of one tablespoon of oil or 25 g of nuts or seeds in your daily diet, and oily fish at least once a week.

- Eat plenty of vitamin- and mineral-rich foods. Each day, include at least five portions of fruits and vegetables; five to eleven portions of grains/starchy vegetables; three portions of low-fat dairy products; and two portions of protein-rich foods (for example, meat, poultry, and legumes).

- Ideally, avoid alcohol for the first 3 months. After that the occasional drink is fine.

- Avoid vitamin A supplements, liver, and liver products.

- Listen to your body and do not exercise if you feel fatigued, nauseous, or dizzy. Do not exercise to the point of exhaustion.

═Further Reading═

National Dairy Council (UK), *Maternal and Fetal Nutrition* (Fact File No. 11, 1994).

British Nutrition Foundation, *Nutrition in Pregnancy* (Briefing Paper, 1994).

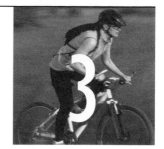

Iron and Sports Anemia

Dr. Eric Watts

Dr. Eric J. Watts, DM, FRCP, MRCPath, Dip Hlth Mgt, is Consultant Hematologist at Basildon Hospital, and his research experience includes the effects of exercise on the blood. He enjoys running and contributes to various sports medicine courses and conferences.

This chapter describes the role of iron in the body, iron balance in women who exercise, and the effects of sports competition on iron status. It also reviews the evidence for or against iron supplementation.

Why Do We Need Iron?

Iron is essential for life. It combines with oxygen, carrying it around the body and into the cells, where energy is released by oxygenating (or burning) the carbon and hydrogen derived from food. Most iron in the blood is in the form of hemoglobin, the material that colors the cells red (see Figure 3.1). The equivalent compound in the muscles is myoglobin.

Although essential for life, iron is also potentially toxic if it is present in excess in certain tissues, especially the heart, liver, and pancreas. Excess iron in the body causes the rare disease of hemochromatosis, which causes patients to develop liver damage, diabetes, and heart failure. The body does not have an effective way of getting rid of excess iron, so it prevents overload by regulating the amount absorbed from the gut, which is normally around 10 percent. With the average Western diet, this is sufficient to supply 1 mg of iron per day, which meets the needs of most men and most nonmenstruating and nonpregnant females. Normally, iron is lost from the body in cells that are shed from the skin and from the gastrointestinal tract, i.e., from the stomach and bowels. Menstruation increases the requirement

3

Table 3.1: *Factors Influencing Iron Absorption*

Absorption is increased by:	Absorption is decreased by:
Ingesting ferrous (heme) iron, e.g., iron found in meat, fish, poultry, and organ meat	Ingesting ferric (nonheme) iron, e.g., iron found in vegetables, legumes, grains, and nuts
The presence of an acidic environment, as in the stomach	The presence of an alkaline environment, as in the duodenum
Vitamin C	Tannin, e.g., tea
Some sugars, e.g., fructose, sorbitol	Phosphates, e.g., egg yolk
An iron-deficient state	Other substances, such as phytate, bran, and inorganic elements such as calcium
Pregnancy	Iron overload
Fasting/dieting	Illness due to infection or inflammation, e.g., arthritis

for iron to the equivalent of 2–3 mg of absorbed iron per day. Women with heavy menstrual periods require more. During pregnancy the requirement for iron is also 2 mg a day (see Table 3.1).

In addition to menstrual-blood loss, blood may be lost through medical conditions such as ulcers or hemorrhoids. When blood is lost from hemorrhoids it is always obvious, but blood can be lost from a duodenal ulcer, which may not cause symptoms, and the blood—being mixed with the other bowel contents—might not be apparent. Hence anemia may often occur without any obvious cause.

What Is Anemia?

Anemia literally means lack of blood. It is normally defined as a condition in which the hemoglobin concentration is insufficient to meet the body's needs. (The normal level of hemoglobin for women is 11.5–16.5 grams per deciliter.) Anemia may also be characterized by a low level of ferritin, which is the storage form of iron. This indicates that iron stores are being depleted. (The normal level of ferritin in the blood is greater than 15 μg per liter.)

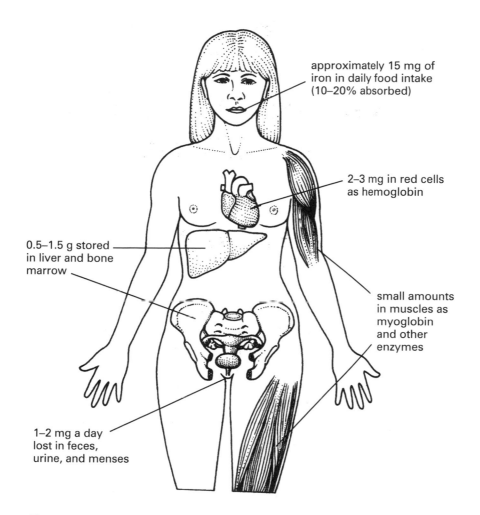

approximately 15 mg of
iron in daily food intake
(10–20% absorbed)

2–3 mg in red cells
as hemoglobin

0.5–1.5 g stored
in liver and bone
marrow

small amounts
in muscles as
myoglobin
and other
enzymes

1–2 mg a day
lost in feces,
urine, and menses

Figure 3.1: *Iron Deposits in the Body*

The characteristic symptoms of anemia are fatigue and breathlessness during exercise. Unfortunately these symptoms are not specific to anemia. Tiredness and fatigue, for example, are very common symptoms in healthy people and can result from stress as well as from physical illness. Anemia may cause poor athletic performance and is worth considering when there is an unexplained loss of form or when training/competition is impaired for some inexplicable reason.

Which Foods Contain Iron?

Foods rich in iron include meat—particularly red meat—poultry, and fish. Although vegetables are not as rich in iron as meat, good vegetable sources are peas and beans (see Table 3.2).

*Practical tip: try to include iron-rich foods (those which are readily absorbed) in your diet **every day**. If you are a vegetarian and do not consume foods with a high bioavailability (i.e., meat, fish, organ meats, etc.), then ensure that you include plenty of nonmeat iron sources. Because the iron in these foods tends to be less readily absorbed, it is important to avoid any practices which further hinder absorption (see Table 3.1). Try also to combine nonmeat sources of iron with vitamin C, since this will improve iron absorption.*

A number of factors affect the absorption of iron. The chemical state of the iron is important: Iron is absorbed more efficiently if it exists in a reduced (or ferrous) form, as it is in meat, poultry, fish, and liver. This is sometimes called heme iron. If it is in the oxidized (or ferric) form, as is found in vegetables, it is absorbed less readily and is known as nonheme iron. It is also absorbed better in an acidic environment, for example, if it is

Table 3.2: *Dietary Sources of Iron*

Iron is well absorbed from (sources offering high bioavailability):	Iron is less well absorbed from (sources offering moderate to low bioavailability):
Meat (especially red meat)	Grains (breakfast cereals, oatmeal, bread, rice, pasta)
Poultry	
Fish	Beans (including baked beans)
Liver and other organ meat	Peas
	Lentils
	Nuts
	Dried fruits (apricots, raisins, dates, prunes)
	Fortified TVP and tofu
	Dark-green leafy vegetables
	Egg yolks
	Molasses

Table 3.3: *The Iron Content of Various Foods*

Food	Iron (mg per portion)	Portion/size
Liver (chicken)	4.75	per 50 g slice
Minced beef (cooked)	3.10	per 100 g portion
Sirloin steak (cooked)	3.80	per large portion (200 g)
Chicken (roasted)	0.8	per four slices
Cod (baked)	0.4	per fillet (100 g)
Mackerel (smoked)	1.20	per small fillet (100 g)
Bran Flakes	6.0	per small bowl (30 g)
Cornflakes	2.0	per small bowl (30 g)
Baked beans	2.8	per half medium can (200 g)
Red kidney beans	4.0	per half medium can (200 g)
Brown bread	1.3	per two average slices
White bread	1.0	per two average slices
Brown rice (raw)	0.7	per 2 oz. portion (uncooked)
White rice (raw)	0.25	per 2 oz. portion (uncooked)
Raisins	1.9	per 2 tablespoons (50 g)
Prunes	2.6	per 10 prunes (100 g)
Dry roasted peanuts	0.5	per small packet (25 g)
Cashew nuts (roasted)	1.6	per small packet (25 g)
Broccoli (boiled)	1.0	per normal portion (40 g)
Cabbage (boiled)	0.3	per 2 large tablespoons (40 g)

taken with lemon or orange juice, which contains ascorbic acid (vitamin C). Certain foods contain substances that form complexes with iron and reduce absorption, for example tea (tannin), chapatis (phytates), and rhubarb (oxalic acid). Meat encourages the absorption of iron by stimulating the stomach to produce acid (see Table 3.1).

The recommended intake of iron (RDA) for adolescent and adult females is either 15 mg or 18 mg (depending on the person's age), but many women do not eat this much. When iron deficiency occurs, the body can increase the proportion of iron absorbed by up to a maximum of 37 percent; this explains why some women who eat less than the RDA are not iron deficient. Iron deficiency is nevertheless very common: researchers from the University of Southampton report that one-third of normal women have no iron stores.

Table 3.3 lists the amount of iron in common foods. Use it to calculate your approximate daily iron intake. *Note: the iron content of different cuts of meat and varying forms of other foods may differ, so use this table only as a rough guide.*

How Do Sports and Exercise Affect Iron Systems?

For the majority of people, sports and exercise have no effect on their iron status, but there are some exceptions. All athletes who undertake endurance training, to the extent that they develop "cardiac conditioning" (a fall in their resting pulse rate), will develop an increase in their blood volume. This can result in a syndrome called sports anemia, in which the hemoglobin concentration falls from the average of 14 to 13.5 grams per deciliter (g/dl). This syndrome is well recognized, and there have been many suggestions as to the cause. Some of the suggestions have led to unnecessary anxiety and concern among exercisers, coaches, and instructors, often leading to unnecessary treatments. It seems paradoxical that when most other physiological measurements show improved function after training, the hemoglobin level should fall, but studies on runners, rowers, cyclists, swimmers, and walkers have consistently shown this to be the case.

What Causes Sports Anemia?

Iron deficiency is often considered to be the cause of sports anemia, and blood loss may occasionally occur in runners. Blood in the urine (hematuria) is particularly easy to detect. It has been reported many times in runners covering distances greater than 10 kilometers (6.2 miles). Investigations with a cystoscope, an instrument which allows the bladder to be inspected from the inside, have shown bruising of the lining of the bladder, presumably as a result of the upper wall of the bladder being repeatedly pressed against the lower wall by the abdominal contents bouncing up and down with each footstrike. Normally the hematuria ceases within hours of completion of a run and the amount of blood loss is seldom significant. One expert has suggested that runners should prevent this from occurring by running with a full bladder—not surprisingly, few runners have taken this advice.

Hemoglobinuria is another well-recognized complication of running or marching. This condition is different from hematuria in that hematuria causes the urine to take on a cloudy appearance, whereas in hemoglobinuria it is clear like rosé wine. Hemoglobinuria occurs in runners who have a very poor style, in particular a high, stomping gait; it also occurs when they run on hard roads, as opposed to grass, bark mulch, or another type of soft trail. There is reason to believe that other activities that involve repetitive foot-strikes, such as high-impact aerobics, can have a similar effect. If it occurs, the exerciser should try to develop a better style. Well-cushioned shoes can also prevent the problem.

Although blood and hemoglobin loss in the urine are well docu-mented, it is highly unlikely that they cause significant iron deficiency. A very small amount of blood can cause marked discoloration of the urine.

Blood loss from the gut during exercise and diarrhea (often referred to as "runner's trots") may also occur, particularly in high-mileage runners or runners who have recently increased their mileage. The cause may be the cumulative effect of repeated minor trauma as the abdominal contents bounce up and down with each footstrike. Alternatively, the bowel may become more permeable or "leaky" as it is starved of oxygen during intense exercise (the blood is diverted away from the gut to the muscles, where more blood is required). After exercise, when the blood returns to the bowel, it may pass through the more permeable bowel wall, where it may cause diarrhea due to an irritant effect. One study in which stool samples were analyzed before and after a marathon showed that the amount of hemoglobin in the stools increased by 30 percent.

Blood loss through the digestive tract may also be increased by the use of anti-inflammatory drugs, such as aspirin and other drugs that may be taken for muscular strains. It is essential to check with your physician before taking any drugs. If they do affect iron absorption, then dietary measures should be taken to compensate for this.

It has been claimed that iron deficiency is common among runners and is the main cause of athletes' anemia. This claim is mainly a result of finding lowered ferritin levels in athletes. Although serum ferritin is normally a good guide to iron stores, it is not reliable in runners. There are many ways to estimate iron stores, but the most accurate is from bone marrow sam-pling, which is unpleasant at best and painful at worst.

Studies have been conducted that analyzed ferritin marrow samples for iron stores in runners and control groups. One such study was performed by B. Magnusson. He investigated 43 middle- and long-distance runners and 119 control subjects, and showed that the athletes had lowered hemoglobin and ferritin levels. From these results one might presume that iron stores were low and anemia likely. However, they all had iron present in their bone marrow, which means that they were *not* iron deficient. He explained the lowered ferritin levels as being due to altered red-cell metabolism in runners, suggesting that more red cells are burst in circulation as a result of footstrike when running, and hence fewer appear in the stores.

Sports anemia is in fact a very misleading term because the syndrome is not a true anemia (in which there is inadequate hemoglobin in the body as a whole). It is rather a consequence of changes that take place as a result of training and is caused by the dilution of the red blood cells by the increased volume of plasma (the watery part of the blood), which is a beneficial adaptation to aerobic exercise. Although measures of hemoglobin and ferritin may appear lower, there is actually the same amount of these substances in total in the body—they have simply been "watered down." Hence, sports anemia is only perceived as a problem if hemoglobin concentration is considered in isolation. It is important to realize that this is simply one adaptation to training that results in improved delivery of oxygen to the tissues. It is clear that this gives an improved, not diminished, athletic performance. So athletes who exhibit sports anemia are not ill; they are actually coping effectively with the stresses of their training load.

This does not mean that sports anemia and iron deficiency anemia may not coexist. The lowered ferritin level in runners makes iron deficiency difficult to diagnose. Every exerciser should check his or her dietary intake of iron. If ferritin levels and dietary levels of iron are low, supplementation with the advice of a physician may be considered.

Sports Anemia and Women Athletes

Even though sports anemia is not a true indication of anemia and iron deficiency, many studies show that female athletes do not consume the RDA for iron of 15 to 18 mg per day. Some females may even consume less than 10 mg per day. Many studies also reveal inadequate calorie intake, possibly as a result of a desire to lose weight. As calorie intake is reduced, so is dietary iron intake, and hence a well-intentioned desire for fitness and weight loss may inadvertently lead to reduced performance due to iron deficiency anemia. Females on very low energy diets (1,500 calories per day) will find it extremely difficult to consume enough iron. This highlights yet another problem of dieting and very low calorie intakes.

It has been claimed, based on the finding of the serum ferritin under 25 μg/l, that up to 80 percent of elite women endurance athletes are iron deficient. This is in my opinion an overestimate, because sports anemia and the dilution of normal levels of ferritin will "mask" the true amount of iron that is stored in the body. These reports have led to concern that athletes who have no iron stores (a condition referred to as latent iron deficiency), but who are not anemic, may suffer from a reduction in performance. A number of studies have investigated this claim by supplementing iron to exercisers who are anemic and to those who have no iron stores but who are not anemic.

It is quite clear that when athletes are genuinely anemic (females with less than 11.5 g/dl hemoglobin), treating them with iron improves their performance. When iron is given to athletes who are not anemic, the majority of studies have not shown any improvement. Some of the studies in which no improvement was seen have been criticized on the basis that not enough iron was given or that the iron was not given for a long enough period of time. Patients who are genuinely iron deficient are normally given ferrous sulfate (200 mg three times a day for 1 month). Studies that use less than this (or that use the equivalent in a different formulation) or that give iron for less than a month cannot claim to have given sufficient iron over a sufficient period of time to test whether the athlete was genuinely iron deficient.

One extremely thorough and notable piece of research was carried out by Newhouse and colleagues in Canada in 1988. They screened 155 female athletes for latent iron deficiency (defined as a hemoglobin level of greater than 12 g/dl but a serum ferritin of lower than 20). The subjects took at least 120 minutes of exercise per week and were mostly recreational runners. On average they did five workouts a week at an average of 40 minutes per workout.

Out of a total of 135 female athletes, they found 40 to have the criteria for latent iron deficiency. They went to great lengths to exclude anybody who had any illness likely to complicate matters, and they carried out a detailed dietary survey as well. They measured fitness through a variety of tests, including an anaerobic speed test and a treadmill test with a progressively increasing workload. They also had samples of the quadriceps (thigh muscle) taken through a needle biopsy in order to investigate the possible effects of tissue iron deficiency.

The volunteers were given either a total of 640 mg of ferrous sulfate per day or a placebo pill. The investigators ensured that the volunteers were in fact taking their pills by counting the number of pills remaining in their bottles after 4 and 8 weeks of study.

After taking iron or placebo for 2 months, the subjects were all reinvestigated. Those given iron showed an increase in the amount of ferritin compared with the placebo group but no increase in total hemoglobin. There were no significant differences in other measurements. The enzyme analysis of the thigh muscle showed no benefit from iron treatment. The mean power and the anaerobic speed test showed no difference in VO_2 max (maximum aerobic capacity). The authors of this study concluded that there was no increase in work capacity (which is the best correlation with athletic performance) and that if there is no anemia, no benefit results from iron treatment.

A particularly important aspect of this work was that a placebo group was included. Some studies which have claimed a benefit from iron treatment have not compared their results with a placebo group. In scientific terms this means that the study which takes in novice recruits and gives them medication in addition to starting them on an exercise program will almost always show very striking improvements in fitness simply because the subjects are embarking upon an exercise program which will improve their health.

An excellent study was carried out in 1971 in Denmark by Vellar and colleagues, who studied new students at a physical education college through the entire academic year. They divided their subjects into three groups: those with low hemoglobin levels, who were given iron; and those with normal levels of hemoglobin, who were divided into placebo and higher supplementation groups. Among their measurements they looked at hemoglobin values and VO_2 max values. As expected, those with low hemoglobin values had improved hemoglobin levels subsequent to treatment with iron. This also increased VO_2 max and endurance performance. However, this may have been a result of their serious training program. The VO_2 max continued to improve during the entire academic year. At the end of the study all three groups showed a great increase in their VO_2 max, but the greatest increase was in the placebo group.

The study therefore showed that the most important requirement for improving endurance capacity is training. Provided that one is not anemic, low iron stores do not appear to be important in terms of athletic performance.

═Summary═

This chapter has presented the case that true anemia is no more common among exercising females than among their sedentary counterparts. The discovery of sports anemia, which is more common, should not be accompanied by panic supplementation. All individuals should follow the recommendations highlighted under the subhead "Practical Points" (on the next page) to ensure that their iron intake is adequate.

Dietary surveys often indicate that females are not consuming the RDA for iron. In the long term, this may put them at increased risk of developing anemia.

Other information we can surmise from studies includes the following:

- True iron deficiency anemia will reduce exercise capacity and negatively affect performance.

- Iron supplementation in females who are anemic will improve blood status and performance.

- Sports anemia is characterized by apparently reduced hemoglobin levels, but performance remains unaffected.

- Sports anemia is mainly the result of the dilution of red blood cells (and therefore hemoglobin levels) caused by an increase in the volume of blood as a result of training.

- Sports anemia masks the true iron status of an individual and sometimes leads to unnecessary iron supplementation.

- Sports anemia should be viewed as a beneficial adaptation to endurance training rather than as an illness or as disadvantageous to performance.

- Females with sports anemia are unlikely to benefit from iron supplementation.

3

<hr>

≡Practical Points≡

- Iron-rich foods (preferably those that are easily absorbed) should be eaten regularly.

- Low-calorie diets should be avoided, as should all restrictive diets that omit major food groups. Such "fad" diets often lead to low iron intake.

- Practices that decrease iron absorption should be avoided.

- Nonmeat (nonheme) sources of iron should be combined with vitamin C to help improve their absorption.

- Vegetarians can obtain adequate quantities of iron from their diet, provided they eat plenty of iron-rich foods and consider the factors that improve their absorption.

- Iron supplements are unnecessary, provided you are consuming plenty of food sources of iron (and are not anemic).

- If you are unsure about your iron status, consult your physician before self-diagnosing supplements. Iron supplements can cause unpleasant side effects.

≡Further Reading≡

L. M. Weight, P. Jacobs, T. D. Noakes, "Dietary Iron Deficiency and Sports Anemia" (*British Journal of Nutrition*, vol. 68, no. 1, July 1992, pp. 253–60).

I. J. Newhouse, D. B. Clement, J. E. Taunton, "The Effects of Prelatent/Latent Iron Deficiency on Physical Work Capacity" (*Medicine, Science, Sports and Exercise*, vol. 21, no. 3, June 1989, pp. 263–8).

E. J. Watts, "Athletes' Anemia" (*British Journal of Sports Medicine*, vol. 23, 1989).

O. D. Vellar, "Physical Performance and Haematological Parameters" (*Acta Medica, Scandinavia*, 522, suppl., 1971, pp. 1–40).

B. Magnusson, "Iron Metabolism and Sports Anemia" (*Acta Medica, Scandinavia*, 216, 1984, pp. 149–55).

W. J. Williams, *Haematology* (McGraw Hill, 2d ed., 1977).

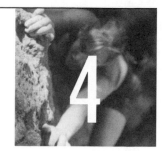

The Menstrual Cycle, Amenorrhea, and Bone Health

Dr. Jane Wilson

Dr. Jane Wilson is a clinical lecturer in rheumatology at the University of Manchester. She was the medical registrar at the British Olympic Centre between 1991 and 1994 and is the Olympic canoe slalom team doctor. She competed for Great Britain in canoe slalom throughout the 1980s and currently competes for Scotland.

During the last two decades it has become recognized that intensive exercise can lead to abnormalities in women's menstrual cycles, and even to the complete cessation of menstrual periods. This may be viewed as a bonus by some athletes, but there may be undesirable short- and long-term consequences. Runners who stop menstruating have lower bone density than their colleagues who have normal periods. In some, bone density is extremely low for their age; this raises the concern that they may be at risk of early osteoporosis (porous bones) and fracture. There is also growing evidence that stress fractures and soft-tissue injuries may be more common in such athletes. Research has helped to define some of the causes of these abnormalities, but many questions still remain.

In order to understand how abnormalities in menstruation result in low bone density, it is necessary to have some knowledge of the physiology of menstruation. This chapter explains how menstruation is controlled in the body, the types of abnormalities that occur in athletes, and factors considered important in the development of menstrual dysfunction. The relationships among bone density, exercise, and menstruation are outlined, and the evidence for menstruation's playing a role in the development of injuries is examined.

What Happens During the Normal Menstrual Cycle?

In Western societies, most girls start to menstruate between the ages of 11 and 15 years, a process called menarche. Although menstrual periods initially may not occur regularly, the normal menstrual cycle becomes established within the first year. The interval between the first day of one period and the first day of the next is surprisingly regular at 28 days, but intervals of 25 to 33 days are also considered to be within normal limits. Blood loss occurs for between 1 and 7 days and is usually less than 80 milliliters. If more than this amount is lost, clots or flooding may occur and the period is considered excessively heavy. Regular menstruation (10–13 cycles per year)

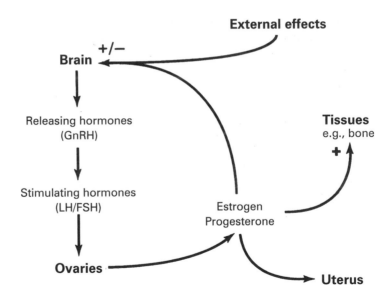

Figure 4.1: *The Menstrual Cycle: The mechanism by which the brain controls hormone production by the ovaries. Estrogen and progesterone in turn act on the brain to control their own production. External influences act on the brain to reduce the production of the releasing hormones.*

> *GnRH = Releasing hormone*
> *LH = Luteinizing hormone*
> *FSH = Follicle-stimulating hormone*

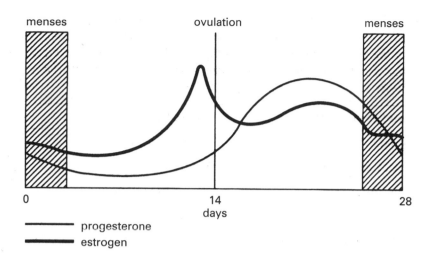

Figure 4.2: *Schematic representation of the changes in blood estrogen and progesterone levels during the 28 day menstrual cycle. If the egg is not fertilized within the first few days of ovulation, the corpus luteum gradually declines and estrogen and progesterone levels fall until at 28 days the lining of the uterus is shed (menstruation).*

is called eumenorrhea, and women with normal menstrual cycles are termed eumenorrheic.

Menstruation is the end result of a complex series of events that start in the brain (see Figure 4.1). "Releasing hormone" (GnRH) is secreted from the hypothalamus in the brain and acts on a second region of the brain (the pituitary), causing the release of two "stimulating hormones": luteinizing hormone (LH) and follicle-stimulating hormone (FSH). These two hormones help to prime the ovaries to produce an egg and then to release it on time. They also cause the ovary to produce the hormones estrogen and progesterone, which act on the uterus to prepare it for the fertilized egg. In addition, estrogen acts on the hypothalamus and pituitary to control the release of FSH and LH so that the whole process is interlocked.

After the release of the egg (ovulation), the ovary forms a yellowish mass of tissue called the corpus luteum—literally "yellow body"—from the ruptured follicle that once held the egg. The corpus luteum secretes further amounts of estrogen and progesterone. If fertilization does not occur, the corpus luteum will die after 14 days, levels of estrogen and progesterone will fall (see Figure 4.2), and the lining of the uterus will be shed (menstruation). The whole cycle then restarts.

Estrogen and progesterone levels vary by as much as 10-fold and 20-fold, respectively, during the cycle and act on other tissues as well as the brain. Of particular importance in the context of this chapter is the influence of these hormones on bone metabolism.

What Abnormalities in the Menstrual Cycle Can Occur?

The menstrual cycle is extremely complex; therefore, it is not surprising that abnormalities can occur. There are many medical causes of menstruation disorders; these are summarized in Table 4.1. Diagnosis of exercise-induced menstrual abnormality can be made only after medical causes have been excluded.

Delayed Menarche

It has been suggested that girls who exercise intensively from a young age start having periods later than average. Certainly in sports such as gymnas-

Table 4.1: Some of the causes of absent menstruation or altered cycle length. The list is not exhaustive, and if further details are required, consultation with a medical professional is advised. The asterisks denote conditions that are relatively common; all the others are either rare or very rare.

Absent menstruation	Altered cycle length
Pregnancy*	Thyroid disorders*
Thyroid disorders*	Eating disorders*
Eating disorders*	Polycystic ovary syndrome*
General illness*	Drugs
Post-Pill (oral contraceptive) amenorrhea*	Hormonal tumors
Polycystic ovary syndrome*	
Ovarian failure, e.g., menopause*	
Removal of ovaries or uterus*	
Drugs	
Imperforate hymen	
Hormonal tumors	
Genetic abnormalities of hormone production	
Chromosomal abnormalities, e.g., Turner's syndrome	

tics there seems to be a predominance of girls who have gone through puberty at a late age. Possibly those who exercise regularly are lighter and have less body fat than their peers; this may delay the onset of periods. One group of researchers postulated that a minimum weight was required before menstruation would start and that 17 percent body fat was necessary for menstruation to be maintained. Others have been unable to confirm these findings.

An alternative explanation is that girls who naturally achieve puberty at a late stage are at an advantage in some sports and therefore continue to compete at a higher level for longer. To date, there are no studies that have followed large populations of children through puberty to determine whether those who are very active do indeed start menstruating later.

Short Cycles (shorter than 25 days)

Athletes, particularly runners, may have shorter menstrual cycles than normal. This is thought to be due to anovulatory cycles, during which an egg is not produced. The consequence of this is that the corpus luteum is not formed, and so the second half of the cycle (the luteal phase) is shorter than 14 days. These cycles are associated with lower than normal levels of estrogen and progesterone.

Long Cycles (more than 35 days)

Many athletes have periods that occur at irregular intervals, for example between 5 and 10 weeks apart. Sometimes a period is missed because of a particularly stressful event, but in most cases they occur at unpredictable times. It is likely that these cycles are also anovulatory and that they are associated with low levels of sex hormones. This condition is termed oligomenorrhea and is usually defined as between four and nine periods a year.

Absent Cycles

Complete loss of menstruation is called amenorrhea, and those who do not menstruate are amenorrheic. Amenorrhea is defined as three or fewer menstrual cycles in 1 year, or no menstrual cycles in 6 months. Blood levels of FSH, LH, estrogen, and progesterone remain at low levels throughout.

Table 4.2: Categorization of Sports According to Whether Low Body Mass May Improve Performance or Increase Scores

Low weight not specific benefit to performance	Low weight likely to improve performance	Performance judged on aesthetic appeal	Competing in weight categories
Heavyweight rowing	Running (middle-	Gymnastics	Judo
Ball games (e.g., soft-	distance, ultra,	Rhythmic gymnastics	Martial arts
ball, soccer, field	cross-country)	Figure skating	Lightweight
hockey, basketball,	Orienteering	Ice dance	rowing
volleyball, tennis)	Race-walking	Dancing (ballet, com-	Wrestling
Golf	Jumping	petitive)	Weightlifting
Sprinting	Pole vault	Bodybuilding	
Field events	Rowing (cox)	Synchronized	
(throwing)	Jockey (flat-racing)	swimming	
Contact sports	Cycling	Diving	
Swimming	Triathlon		
Water polo	Climbing		
Skiing	(competitive)		
Speed skating	Windsurfing		
Luge/bobsled	(Olympic)		
	Sailing (some classes)		

What Are the Causes of Menstrual Disorder in Athletes?

The rate of menstrual disorders in athletes varies from 1 percent to more than 50 percent, whereas in the population as a whole it is approximately 3–5 percent. The condition is more common in sports in which low weight in some way conveys an advantage to the competitor (see Table 4.2).

Low weight for height improves times in distance runners, and ice skaters have been shown to jump higher when they have a low weight-to-height ratio. In gymnastics, ballet, ice skating, and ice dancing, performance is judged partly on the aesthetic appeal of the athlete, and "thinness" may be an advantage. In this group of athletes, estimates of menstrual irregularities are nearly all greater than 25 percent. At risk too are competitors who have to conform to a certain weight category. Some of these athletes may compete well below their natural weight.

These observations have focused attention on the role of weight and body composition in the development of menstrual disorders—and indeed these appear to be key elements. Usually it is the accumulation of a number of risk factors that precipitates the change. Figure 4.3 shows a number of factors that appear to be related to menstrual dysfunction; some of these are discussed in more detail below. But how do these various factors cause disruption in the physiological processes involved in menstruation? Studies on the hormonal changes in athletic amenorrhea have shown that the hypothalamus is where the abnormalities start. By an unknown mechanism, the hypothalamus is inhibited from producing the correct amount of releasing hormone. This in return reduces the production of LH and FSH from the pituitary, and so the ovary is not stimulated to prepare an egg for release. The corpus luteum is not formed, and levels of estrogen and progesterone remain low throughout the cycle.

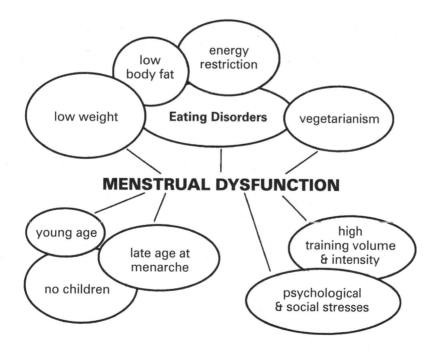

Figure 4.3: *Nonmedical factors likely to contribute to the development of menstrual irregularity in athletes. Women with the greatest number of risk factors are most likely to develop oligomenorrhea.*

Training Volume

There is a strong relationship between the volume of training and the incidence of irregular periods in runners. In one study an almost linear relationship between the number of miles run per week and the prevalence of amenorrhea was found. Approximately 28 percent of those running 40 miles per week had amenorrhea, whereas nearly 45 percent of those running 80 miles per week were affected. In the same study sedentary women, matched for age, had only a 2 percent incidence of amenorrhea. Similar values have been found by other research workers.

At present it is not known whether it is only the *volume* of training that is important or whether the *intensity* of training has an additional effect. It is also unknown whether it is possible to avoid this undesirable effect of high mileage by cross-training with cycling, swimming, or other training modalities. Research is eagerly awaited in this field.

Body Composition

In the study quoted above, the relationship between miles run per week and amenorrhea held true even when the athletes were split according to weight category. However, those athletes who weighed less than 50 kg (110 pounds) were twice as likely to be amenorrheic than those weighing more than 50 kg. Weight thus appears to be of great significance in this equation.

Many studies show that amenorrheic athletes weigh less and have less body fat and a lower weight-to-height ratio than athletes with normal cycles. Although not all researchers agree with these findings, anecdotal reports are common in which the athlete acknowledges that when her weight drops below a certain value she ceases to menstruate. The weight at which this occurs is specific for each athlete and might partially explain why not all research is in agreement on this issue.

Energy Restriction and Eating Disorders

Most athletes do not need to diet in order to maintain optimum weight, but some pay particular attention to calorie intake and restrict food consumption to very low levels. In many, the urge to diet is based on erroneous beliefs that they are too fat. In one study of teenage American swimmers, 17.9 percent of underweight girls and 60.5 percent of average-weight girls were inappropriately trying to lose weight. Restriction of calories may be implicated in the development of amenorrhea: analysis of ten recently published papers reveals that amenorrheic runners consume an average of 300 calories per day less than eumenorrheic runners (1,737 calories/day versus 2,026 calories/day). It is tempting to suppose that there is a minimum energy intake required by the body for basic physiological functions to occur, but as yet a direct link between low energy intake and menstrual abnormality has not been proven.

Not only do athletes restrict calories, they may also develop full eating disorders such as anorexia nervosa and bulimia nervosa, both of which are well known to be associated with abnormal menstruation. (These disorders are covered in Chapter 8 and will therefore not be discussed in great depth here.) A recent study carried out at the British Olympic Medical Center on 50 national and international middle- and long-distance runners found that 50 percent of the amenorrheic athletes had either subclinical or clinical eating disorders, whereas only 12 percent of the eumenorrheic runners were affected. Similar results have been obtained by other workers in a variety of sports. A combination of psychological stresses and insufficient calorie intake can also cause menstrual disruption.

Vegetarianism

In several studies carried out on runners, a higher incidence of vegetarianism was noted in those with irregular periods. However, all of these papers involved very small numbers of athletes. In nonathletic women, vegetarian weight-reducing diets can induce menstrual irregularities such as loss of ovulation or amenorrhea. This may be an area of fruitful research in the future, but at present only cautious conclusions should be drawn.

Previous Menstrual History

Women who have had a late menarche or who have had previous menstrual irregularity are more likely to develop oligomenorrhea or amenorrhea if they start to train intensively. Conversely, women seem less likely to develop irregular periods with training after they have had children. Even athletes who have had prolonged amenorrhea prior to pregnancy may have completely regular periods afterwards, despite intensive training. This may be due to increases in weight or body fat but may also represent changes occurring at the hypothalamic level.

Psychological Stress

It is well recognized that women from all walks of life can stop having periods during times of stress. In the life of a young athlete there are often many conflicting stresses such as school or college work, exams, boyfriends, qualification races, and family pressures. A combination of these may be sufficient to interrupt the menstrual cycle for a short time.

Can Amenorrheic Women Become Pregnant?

Many active women are concerned that prolonged amenorrhea means they are infertile. This is not the case. It is even possible to conceive a baby before having a period. This is because the ovary produces the egg when the lining of the uterus is primed, and it is only if the egg is not fertilized that the lining is shed (menstruation). Therefore, be warned that contraception must be practiced even when a woman is not menstruating!

Exercise, Sex Hormones, and Bone Density

How Does Exercise Affect Bone Strength?

Bone is not an inert substance that, once formed, stays the same for life. Instead, it is in a constant state of turnover so that old bone is removed and new bone is laid down. This enables bone to maintain its strength and to adapt to changes in its environment. In particular, bone responds to mechanical tension so that new bone is built up in places of maximum strain (for example, in the legs of a runner, the forearm of a tennis player, or the lumbar spine of a rower). Exercise therefore has beneficial effects on the skeleton by promoting strong bones with a higher than normal bone density.

It is not surprising, then, to find that bone density is higher in women who undertake regular exercise than in sedentary women of the same age. At the British Olympic Medical Centre, researchers have shown that female runners with regular periods have very much higher bone density in their hips than the average European woman, even in athletes approaching menopause. If this increase in bone density is maintained into older age, these women will be at reduced risk of osteoporosis and hip fractures.

Are Sex Hormones Important in Bone Health?

In women the hormones estrogen and progesterone act directly on bone cells to maintain the bone-turnover cycle. When levels of these hormones are low (as in athletic amenorrhea), resorption of old bone proceeds without check while new bone formation is reduced. The overall result is loss of bone mineral and thinning of the microscopic framework on which new bone is built.

How Does Bone Density Change with Age?

Bone density increases rapidly during the pubertal years and reaches a peak around age 30 (see Figure 4.4). From the age of about 35, there is a gradual decline in bone density of 0.5 percent to 1.0 percent per year until menopause. At menopause, estrogen and progesterone fall to very low levels, and there is a rapid loss of bone mineral (up to 8 percent per year) for several years. Gradually, bone adapts to the new levels of hormones, and

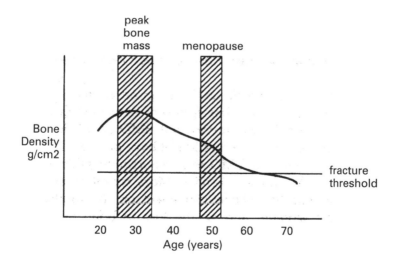

Figure 4.4: *Schematic representation of changes in bone mineral density with age in normal women. Bone density rises rapidly through the pubertal years, reaches a peak in the third and fourth decades, and then declines slowly. There is a period of 3–8 years after menopause when bone loss is more rapid because of falling estrogen and progesterone levels. The fracture threshold is a theoretical level below which osteoporotic fractures are likely to occur. This level is reached in the mid-sixties in the average woman. Those with above-average bone density will cross the fracture threshold at a later age, and those with below-average bone density will be at risk before they are 60 years old.*

the rate of loss slows to about 1 percent per year. It is after menopause, therefore, that women become at risk for osteoporosis and fractures. Sites at particular risk of fracture are the wrist, spine, and hip.

Peak bone mass (i.e., the maximum achieved during a lifetime) is to some extent determined by the genetic make-up of the individual, but it can be increased by regular exercise and decreased by immobility, chronic illness, smoking, some drugs, and of course low levels of sex hormones. It may be possible to slow down the age-related loss of bone mineral by exercise and hormone replacement therapy. The lifetime risk of osteoporotic fracture is related to peak bone mass; the higher it is, the less likely an individual is to ever suffer from osteoporosis. In amenorrheic athletes the concern is that they may never achieve their maximum potential bone mass and may therefore develop osteoporosis early in life and have a greater risk of fractures.

Do Amenorrheic Women Have a Lower Bone Density?

Much of the initial work on bone mineral density (BMD) in athletes compared the lumbar spines of eumenorrheic and amenorrheic runners. It was found that BMD could be as much as 25 percent lower in runners who did not have periods. However, this tells us little about how BMD in amenorrheic athletes compares with that of women who do not exercise. More recent work shows that running has little beneficial effect on the lumbar spine in amenorrheic women, and so the loss in bone mineral due to low estrogen levels is marked (see Figure 4.5). In some amenorrheic women, bone density can be as much as 30 percent lower than the average for their age and might be the equivalent of a 70-year-old woman. Two studies show a linear relationship between the number of periods per year and the bone density—the fewer the periods, the lower the density. This is also demonstrated in Figure 4.5.

Rowers are known to have strong back muscles, and it is interesting to note that BMD of the lumbar spine in a group of elite rowers has been found to be much higher than in either a group of sedentary women or a group of elite long-distance runners. This highlights the site-specific effect of exercise on bone.

While running appears to have little effect on the BMD of the lumbar spine, *hip* BMD has been shown to be high in eumenorrheic runners.

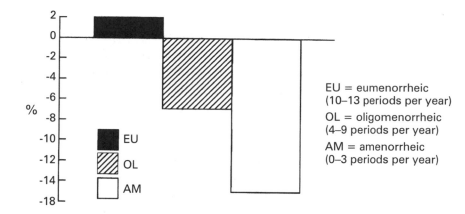

Figure 4.5: *Bone density of the lumbar spine of middle- and long-distance runners ages 17–35, expressed as a percentage of the average for an age-matched normal population. Note the linear relationship between the number of periods per year and the bone density. The bone density of eumenorrheic runners is not significantly different from the average population, but that of both oligomenorrheic and amenorrheic groups are significantly lower than expected for their age.*

(From work undertaken at the British Olympic Medical Centre)

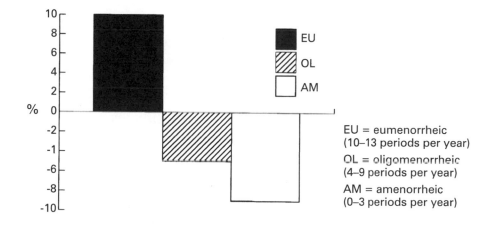

Figure 4.6: *Bone density of the left hip of middle- and long-distance runners ages 17–35, expressed as a percentage of the average for an age-matched normal population. Note the linear relationship between the number of periods per year and the bone density. The bone density of eumenorrheic runners is significantly greater than that of the average population, and that of the amenorrheic group is significantly lower than expected.*

(From work undertaken at the British Olympic Medical Centre)

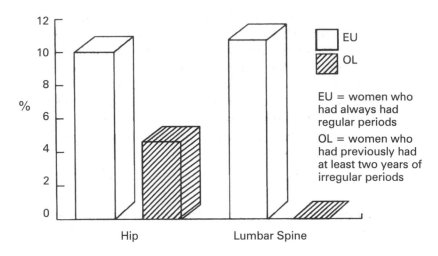

Figure 4.7: *Bone density of the left hip of premenopausal middle- and long-distance runners age 40 and over, expressed as a percentage of the average for an age-matched normal population. There is a significant difference between the two groups in the BMD of the lumbar spine but not at the hip. This suggests long-term effects of menstrual irregularity on bone density that might have been partially offset by return of menstruation and continued exercise.*

(From work undertaken at the British Olympic Medical Centre)

Therefore, running may be a sufficient stimulus to prevent bone loss at this site. Some data suggest that there is indeed preservation of bone in the hip of runners, but researchers at the BOMC have found that amenorrheic athletes have considerable bone loss here despite intensive training (see Figure 4.6).

What Are the Long-Term Consequences of a Low Bone Mineral Density?

Only a few studies have attempted to answer this question. It appears that if menstruation returns, or if the athlete takes estrogen therapy, bone density increases by approximately 4–5 percent in the first year. It is unknown whether such an increase is sustained over the following years, but data from postmenopausal women who have been treated with hormone replacement therapy suggests that in the second year the gain is less. From the third year onwards bone density is maintained but does not increase further. An overall increase of 8–10 percent may therefore be expected.

But the future may not be too bleak for amenorrheic athletes. In one study on premenopausal veteran runners age 40 and over who had

had menstrual irregularity in the past, BMD was found to be close to or higher than the population average for that age group. Although bone density of the lumbar spine was significantly lower than in a comparable group of veteran runners who had always had regular periods, BMD of the hip was just as high (see Figure 4.7). This might mean that when menstruation returns, BMD increases and is then maintained because of the beneficial effects of exercise. To determine whether this applies to all women with amenorrhea, long-term studies are required which follow women runners from their teens to menopause at least.

Do Amenorrheic Women Have More Muscle and Tendon Injuries?

There are many anecdotal reports of runners who seem to have frequent soft-tissue injuries. Many of these runners do not have regular periods. Studies on both runners and dancers have found a higher frequency of soft-tissue injuries in those with irregular periods. It is unclear why this is so, although estrogen does have some effect on tendons and ligaments. For instance, just prior to giving birth—when estrogen levels are very high—the mother's ligaments become supple and stretch readily. This enables the pelvis to widen to allow the birth of the child. It is possible that the opposite applies in athletes: that when estrogen levels are very low, ligaments become less supple and more susceptible to injury.

Are Stress Fractures More Common in Women with Menstrual Irregularity?

Several reports have shown an increased incidence of stress fractures in athletes with menstrual irregularity. Initially it was postulated that this is due to low bone density, but subsequent studies have not confirmed this. An alternative explanation may be that adequate estrogen levels are required for the normal bone-turnover cycle. If estrogen levels are low, bone adaptation is slowed and microfractures occur more readily or heal more slowly. Again, further research is required in this area.

The full bone-turnover cycle takes about three months, and major changes in training techniques should therefore be planned gradually over at least 10 weeks. If training is altered too rapidly, microscopic fractures can occur in bone; if these are not allowed to heal they can ultimately lead to a stress fracture. A typical example is that of a long-distance runner who returned to training after injury and aimed to reach her previous level of 50 miles per week within 6 weeks. Four to 8 weeks after training started, she had gradual onset of pain in her shin, and a stress fracture was diagnosed.

Is There a Greater Risk of Osteoporotic Fractures?

There are several reports of stress fractures leading to complete fractures, but only recently has there been a report of an osteoporotic-type fracture occurring in a young athlete. In the case reported, a 30-year-old long-distance runner with a history of 7 years of athletic amenorrhea was known to have bone density below the lower limit of normal for her age. She had had several stress fractures, and while she was recovering from one of these she slipped at the swimming pool and fractured her upper arm. The type of fracture sustained was that commonly seen in postmenopausal women with osteoporosis.

It is perhaps surprising that more athletes with low bone density do not sustain osteoporotic fractures. It is possible that, although bone density is similar to that of older women, there is less damage to the microscopic framework. This allows the bone to withstand greater forces before fractures occur. It is also possible that, because the microscopic framework is still intact, recovery from low bone density is more likely in the young athlete compared to the 70-year-old woman. These questions have not yet been answered.

How Can Athletic Amenorrhea Be Treated?

Although many questions remain about the long-term consequences of amenorrhea, current opinion is that it should be investigated and treated (if appropriate) when it lasts for longer than 6 months. A general practitioner will be able to exclude many of the common causes of menstrual disorder, but full assessment and management will require referral to a specialist with an interest in this field. Such doctors may be gynecologists, endocrinologists, bone specialists, or sports physicians. Other specialists may also need to be consulted, such as sports nutritionists, exercise physiologists, psychologists, and psychiatrists. Investigation will entail detailed histories, physical examination, blood tests, and in some cases special scans. If amenorrhea is prolonged it is appropriate to measure bone density of the lumbar spine and/or hip.

Treatment with hormones may not be necessary if risk factors such as low weight, eating disorders, and overtraining can be reduced so that menstruation is resumed. However, many athletes are unwilling to reduce training or to gain weight, and if amenorrhea continues despite reduction of all other risk factors, hormone therapy is usually prescribed. Precisely which hormone preparation is used will depend on individual circumstances and the preference of the specialist. Both the estrogen-containing oral contraceptive pill (OCP) and hormone replacement therapy (HRT) are likely to reduce further loss of bone mineral and may slightly increase bone density.

Hormone replacement therapy is designed to replace estrogen and progesterone in physiological amounts in postmenopausal women. The amount of each type of hormone may not therefore suit all premenopausal women, but the advantage is that they are "natural" hormones and therefore have fewer side effects on the blood than the OCP (the OCP contains synthetic estrogen and progesterone in relatively large amounts; this suppresses the normal menstrual cycle by preventing the release of LH and FSH by the brain). Side effects common to both forms of treatment include weight gain, breast tenderness, breakthrough bleeding, and emotional upset, but most of these settle down after the first few months of treatment. It is important to realize that millions of women worldwide take both types of treatment without any side effects whatsoever.

Calcium supplementation has been suggested as an alternative to hormone therapy, but at the moment there is no evidence to show that it prevents the loss of bone mineral in athletic amenorrhea. Certainly calcium supplementation *in addition to* hormone therapy is a sensible approach, particularly as the diet of some athletes is low in this essential mineral.

Hormone treatment can continue for many years until the athlete decides to reduce training or start a family. In most cases, normal menstruation returns within a matter of months. Failure to start menstruating within a year suggests that there are other causes of menstrual disorder such as a medical problem, a persistent eating disorder, or low body weight. In a few women, special hormone therapy will help to "kick start" the system. A flowchart for the suggested management of athletic amenorrhea is given in Figure 4.8.

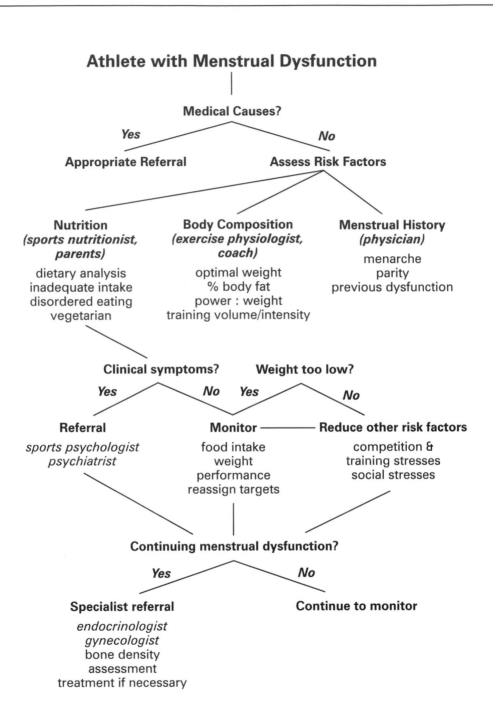

Athlete with Menstrual Dysfunction

Medical Causes?

Yes — Appropriate Referral

No — Assess Risk Factors

Nutrition
(sports nutritionist, parents)

dietary analysis
inadequate intake
disordered eating
vegetarian

Body Composition
(exercise physiologist, coach)

optimal weight
% body fat
power : weight
training volume/intensity

Menstrual History
(physician)

menarche
parity
previous dysfunction

Clinical symptoms?   Weight too low?

Yes — Referral   *No*   *Yes*   *No*

Referral

sports psychologist
psychiatrist

Monitor ——— **Reduce other risk factors**

food intake
weight
performance
reassign targets

competition &
training stresses
social stresses

Continuing menstrual dysfunction?

Yes — **Specialist referral**   *No* — **Continue to monitor**

endocrinologist
gynecologist
bone density
assessment
treatment if necessary

Figure 4.8: Suggested flowchart for the assessment and management of menstrual dysfunction in athletes. Specialists who may be able to provide help at each stage are shown in italics.

═Case History═

- A 14-year-old runner was told by one of her "friends" that her tummy stuck out. She decided to diet and lost 7 pounds. It made no difference to her shape, but she ran faster. This encouraged her to lose more weight, and again she ran faster. She now weighed 98 pounds and was winning races. She felt good, and people were starting to talk about her achievements on the track. So she lost more weight. She felt guilty every time she ate, so she made sure she always felt "empty" by vomiting after meals. Her weight dropped to 84 pounds.

- By now she was training at least twice a day and felt exhausted all the time. However, she still "knew" that she was fat and had to lose more weight. She developed a stress fracture.

- When she got down to 70 pounds she was admitted to an adolescent psychiatric unit for management of her anorexia and bulimia. Two years later her eating habits were improving, but she still had not had any periods and had endured three stress fractures. She was referred to a hormone specialist who started her on treatment. One year later she had nearly conquered her eating problems, weighed 98 pounds, and was starting to run well again. Bone density measurements at this stage revealed her to be 10 percent below average for her age.

═Practical Points═

- Exercise increases bone mineral density (BMD). Generally, active women have a higher bone density and lower risk of osteoporosis than sedentary women.

- Menstrual problems such as oligomenorrhea (irregular periods) and amenorrhea (absent periods) are more common in women involved in sports where a low body weight and low body fat are considered advantageous, for example, in long-distance running, gymnastics, and figure skating.

- There is no single cause of amenorrhea; rather, a combination of factors are responsible. These include high training volume and possibly intensity, psychological stress, low body-fat levels, low body weight, calorie restriction, late age at menarche, and disordered eating.

- Subclinical and clinical eating disorders are more common among exercisers with amenorrhea compared with those with normal periods.

- Bone mineral density is significantly lower in amenorrheic athletes compared with athletes with normal periods. The BMD may be up to 30 percent lower than average for their age, despite intense training.

- There is a linear relationship between number of periods per year and BMD: the fewer the number of periods, the lower the BMD.

- Once normal menstrual cycles return, BMD increases.

- Amenorrheic athletes have a greater risk of soft-tissue injuries, stress fractures, and early osteoporosis.

- Amenorrhea may be reversed and normal periods established by increasing body weight, reducing training volume and intensity, and ensuring normal eating patterns.

- If amenorrhea fails to respond to the above strategy, hormone replacement therapy or estrogen-containing oral contraceptive pills may be prescribed.

- If you suffer from irregular periods (between four and nine periods/year) or absent periods (less than three periods/year or no periods in 6 months), reduce the risk of stress fractures and early osteoporosis by:

    – gradually reducing training frequency, volume, and intensity

    – changing your training program to include more cross-training

    – eating a little more to put on some weight—gradually

    – not overly restricting your calorie or food intake

    – consulting your doctor, who will refer you to a dietitian, sports nutritionist, sports psychologist, or a self-help group if you suspect you may have an eating disorder

    – taking steps to reduce your mental and emotional stress

    – taking a temporary break from competition to reduce the stress from a busy competitive schedule.

- If menstrual irregularities continue despite your taking these measures, ask your doctor to refer you to a specialist.

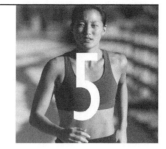

Nutrition for Team Sports

John Brewer

John Brewer, B.Sc., MPhil, is Head of the Human Performance Centre at Lilleshall National Sports Centre, specializing in the provision of sports science support to athletes, particularly those involved in team sports. He has worked with the England cricket team and the England soccer team and published a number of academic papers.

The introduction of national sports leagues and international competitions for women has meant that female participation in team sports has grown at both the elite and the grassroots levels. In 1990, the first women's soccer World Cup was held in the U.S., and in 1994 England became the winner of the second women's rugby World Cup. Since such competitions often attract a high media profile, it is inevitable that more and more women will be encouraged to participate; however, many of the governing bodies of these fledgling sports are still small and have relatively poor coach-education structures, and so advice in such areas as sports nutrition is relatively limited. It is absolutely essential that correct information and practical advice be given to both coaches and competitors at an early stage to ensure that the athletes remain healthy and the sports continue to develop successfully.

What Is the Link Between Team Sports and Nutrition?

Considerable research links correct nutritional practices with success in individual sports such as cycling, swimming, and running. Researchers show, for example, that high amounts of carbohydrate in the diet can lead to direct improvements in running or cycling performance. This knowledge has encouraged many male and female competitors in individual sports to consume high-carbohydrate diets as a means to improve their performance.

Unfortunately, the link between correct nutrition and performance in team sports is much harder to demonstrate. This is because success in team sports depends on many factors, including skill, strategy (tactics), and teamwork, as well as fitness and diet. Because of these different factors, it is often much harder to convince coaches and competitors in team sports that correct nutrition is as important for them as it is for those involved in individual sports.

A number of research studies undertaken in the 1990s show that with correct nutrition, higher work rates can be sustained for longer periods during sports such as soccer and hockey—particularly during the second half of the game—while recovery rates after matches are also improved. The characteristic fatigue experienced in the second half can be alleviated if the player consumes a carbohydrate-rich diet prior to the competition. Correct nutrition does not guarantee success however; it is only one of the contributing factors that can help improve the performance of both individuals and the team as a whole.

What Do Players Currently Eat?

To date, very little research has been done to assess the nutritional habits of female games players. However, a recent study of female hockey players found that their diets consisted of 54 percent carbohydrate, 27 percent fat, and 15 percent protein. It also found that during the playing season, energy intake appeared to be lower than energy expenditure. Somewhat alarmingly, eight out of nine players involved in the study were found to be attempting to lose weight during the playing season; the calcium and iron intake of these players was 30 percent below the recommended daily intake.

In a similar study of female basketball players, energy intake values were found to be lower than estimated energy expenditure, while in many other sports there are reports that females appear to be maintaining high training loads on a lower caloric intake than might be expected. If this really is the case, then the athletes should be losing body weight. However, several studies report that the athletes' weight generally remains stable, despite the reported discrepancy in energy intake versus energy expenditure. The current scientific consensus is that there is no strange metabolic adaptation to low energy intake; there is simply a tendency for female athletes to under-report their food intake! The main problem with such low-calorie diets is that they can result in a low intake of vitamins, minerals, protein, and carbohydrate.

While the available evidence is somewhat limited, there are clear indications that many female athletes should increase their carbohydrate intake in order to sustain intensive training and competition. However, it should be recognized that some individuals will attempt to reduce their caloric intake in order to decrease body weight, so maximum sensitivity should be used when advising female athletes on their nutritional practices. Persons who are concerned about their body weight should be made aware that, with careful thought and planning, a high-carbohydrate diet can be consumed without any increase in total energy intake.

What Are the Dietary Recommendations for Team Players?

In 1991, the International Olympic Committee (IOC) produced a series of recommendations for sports nutrition for both male and female athletes in all sports. It suggested that the diet of an active athlete should consist of between 60 and 70 percent of total energy intake from carbohydrate, 15 percent of total energy intake from protein, and no more than 30 percent of total energy intake from fat. (For practical advice on how to achieve these goals, see Chapter 1.)

It also suggested that—provided their food intake was sufficient in terms of both quality and quantity—there should be no need for female athletes to take vitamin or mineral supplements. In 1994, the world govern-ing body for soccer, FIFA, accepted that the recommendations of the IOC also applied to female soccer players, and advised all women involved in team sports to pay particular attention to their intake of iron and calcium.

What Happens If Energy Intake Is Too Low?

The recommendations of the IOC only referred to an appropriate carbohy-drate intake based on a percentage of total energy intake. Many researchers who have worked with female competitors in team sports have noted that a number of athletes consume diets that have a low total energy intake. For these women, even a high percentage intake of carbohydrate will still result in a low absolute carbohydrate intake. It has been concluded that low total energy intakes are often due to the fact that some females restrict their total energy intake to control body weight at the expense of consuming an adequate energy intake to supply them with the fuel they need for training and competing. In severe cases this can lead to eating disorders, menstrual dysfunction, and loss of bone minerals (in particular, calcium).

Eating disorders that result in bone mineral decalcification have been linked to increased incidence of stress fractures in female athletes (see Chapter 4). While it is unlikely that females involved in team sports will cover the same total distances as many female endurance athletes, the stresses and rotational forces experienced in many team sports place severe demands on the bones and joints. It is therefore safe to assume that low energy intakes combined with possible disordered eating patterns could well lead to an increased risk of injuries and stress fractures in female competitors in team sports.

However, it should be pointed out that the probable incidence of eating disorders among team-sports players is likely to be far lower than that found in individual sportswomen where body-fat levels are deemed to be crucial. In team sports, a low body-fat percentage is not necessarily seen as a primary factor influencing performance, and therefore these athletes are probably far less likely to drastically reduce their total energy intake. Nevertheless, those involved in advising female team-sports competitors about their diets should be aware of the potential existence of this problem and, indeed, take every care to ensure that their advice does not cause females to restrict their energy intake. This is a particular concern when advising on areas such as weight loss.

How Much Carbohydrate Is Recommended?

Recommendations regarding the amount of carbohydrate that female games players should consume should be based on the total energy intake of each individual. For those who consume more than 45 calories/kg per day, a minimum of 55 percent of total energy intake should come from carbohydrate. However, for females who are consuming less than 45 calories/kg per day, carbohydrate consumption should be based on a minimum of 6 g/kg per day. (To determine body weight in kilograms, divide weight in pounds by 2.2). This ensures that those people who have a low total energy intake are at least getting a large proportion of that energy from carbohydrate.

Use either of the tables below as a rough guide for calculating how much carbohydrate you need.

Table 5.1: *Recommended Carbohydrate Consumption for Females Participating in Team Sports*

Weight	Carbohydrate (g)
50 kg (110 pounds)	300
60 kg (132 pounds)	360
70 kg (154 pounds)	420
80 kg (176 pounds)	480

Table 5.2: *Fifty-Five Percent of Total Energy Intake Should Come from Carbohydrate*

Calories	5 percent of energy (calories)	Amount of carbohydrate (g)
2,000	1,100	275
2,500	1,375	345
3,000	1,650	415
3,500	1,925	480
4,000	2,200	550

Long-Term Nutritional Strategies

It is important that female athletes receive nutritional advice that encompasses the whole of the 12-month competitive cycle and not just the playing season. During the off-season period, many athletes use significantly less energy due to the fact that their training load is reduced. It is therefore essential that during this phase of the season players make a conscious effort to decrease their energy intake to avoid increasing their body-fat levels. This can be achieved by consuming less food in total but keeping the nutrient balance the same—still consuming plenty of carbohydrate and moderate quantities of fat, protein, and alcohol, but smaller meals and snacks.

If body fat is allowed to increase during the off-season, players face the prospect of having to lose weight during the preseason period. This can often result in extreme dieting and restricted energy intakes to levels that are below energy output during a time when training intensity is extremely high. The player will suffer from fatigue and an inability to train consistently during a period when training is essential. If the athlete needs to lose weight

5

during this time, then the fat content of the diet should be reduced. It is essential that the carbohydrate intake remain high and that the athlete continue to consume high-carbohydrate meals and snacks if she is to continue to train while losing weight.

Short-Term Nutritional Strategies

It is vitally important to remember that a high-carbohydrate diet is needed to support training as well as games and tournaments. Female athletes must be encouraged to eat high levels of carbohydrate on a 7-day-a-week basis and not simply during the short-term buildup before important games; they should be reminded that carbohydrate is the key substrate for the provision of energy. They should also be counseled on the vital role that a balanced diet can play, both with regard to the provision of energy and to the prevention and maintenance of general health and well-being.

In individual sports it is common for competitors to gear their training and preparation for specific *peaks* that may occur only once or twice during the competitive season. However, in team sports such as softball, soccer, and basketball, games are played at regular intervals throughout a season, often with equal importance. If a team attempts to peak for the finals of a cup competition, there is a chance that it will get knocked out in the first round. Attempting to peak for team sports therefore presents the coach and competitor with very different problems than those encountered by people involved in individual sports; teams need to be able to produce a series of peaks at regular intervals throughout the season. A correct nutritional strategy is fundamental to achieving this.

How Can Diet Support Regular Games?

Peaking for the next game should start immediately after the current game is completed: players should be encouraged to consume carbohydrate-rich foods and fluids immediately after each game. This is because the enzymes responsible for the conversion of carbohydrate into glycogen work most efficiently during the early postexercise phase. Consuming carbohydrate in liquid or solid form soon after exercise accelerates recovery rates and improves the ability of competitors to train or play again within a relatively short period of time. Most players will benefit from consuming 50–100 g of carbohydrate immediately after a game, and another high-carbohydrate

Table 5.3: *Postgame Snacks*

The following foods/drinks contain approximately 50 g of carbohydrates:
3 medium-sized bananas
3 tablespoons raisins
1½ Pop Tarts
large handful hard candies
4 large handfuls caramel popcorn
1½ bagels or muffins
banana sandwich
750 ml "isotonic" sports drink, i.e., Gatorade, Powerade
600 ml orange juice (just over a pint)

meal about 2 hours later. Coaches should try to make carbohydrate-rich foods available in the locker room after a match; and for away matches carbohydrate rich food should also be provided during the journey both to and from games. Table 5.3 suggests some ideal snacks in 50 g carbohydrate portions for consumption immediately after a game. Remember that if food is not tolerated during this time, drinks that contain carbohydrate can be used instead.

Game Preparation

Players should follow a carbohydrate-rich diet in the week prior to a match; they should also ensure that they maintain hydration by drinking water regularly.

The pregame meal should be high in carbohydrate and relatively low in protein, fat, and fiber (unless the individual is sure that she can tolerate high-fiber foods at this time). This meal will typically be consumed 2–3 hours prior to the start of the game. Ideas for the pregame meal are discussed in Chapter 9.

During the Game

During the game, sports drinks are ideal because they meet the twin aims of supplying carbohydrates and fluid. These should preferably be consumed at frequent intervals. It is usually recommended that 300–600 ml of fluid be ingested immediately prior to a game, for two main reasons:

- to preempt sweat losses in the first half of the game

- because fluid is absorbed into the bloodstream more quickly if there is a greater quantity in the stomach

Some players may not be able to tolerate a large quantity of fluid immediately before exercise. They should practice in training and aim to consume as much liquid as is comfortable prior to a game, "topping this up" during suitable breaks in play.

At halftime, players should choose sports drinks rather than tea or sliced oranges. This will ensure that they continue to replace lost fluid and will provide extra energy. Tea contains caffeine, a diuretic, and is therefore potentially dehydrating. Oranges contain only small amounts of fluid and carbohydrate—large quantities would have to be consumed to influence fluid or carbohydrate status.

How Do Women Fit Proper Nutrition into Their Day?

While women in many countries are now beginning to compete in a wider variety of team sports, in the vast majority of cases this competition is on a part-time or amateur basis. Very rarely are females able to devote themselves to full-time training and competition. This means that their sport has to be combined with full-time occupations, and training or games have to be fitted in during recreational time. This immediately presents problems for the preparation and consumption of meals, particularly since in most countries women are responsible for the preparation and cooking of food. The tendency to miss meals or to eat only in limited amounts is therefore increased.

Females involved in team sports should be encouraged to eat small, high-carbohydrate meals at regular intervals throughout the day, especially if they are likely to experience difficulty in obtaining a main meal. Increased responsibility will rest with the partner or family of the athlete to provide suitable meals for her after she has completed her training or playing during the evenings and on weekends. In many societies this may require a change in traditional roles.

Individual Preferences

A good coach will be aware that the training needs of her team members vary from one individual to another. The same is also true of nutritional needs.

While the general principles of good sports nutrition apply to the whole team, the coach should be aware that individuals within the squad will have their own personal tastes and preferences and that these must be considered when she advises them on their diet. A global nutritional strategy that does not take these aspects into account will almost certainly result in many individuals paying little or no attention to what the coach says about nutrition. It is therefore essential that individual consultations take place to determine each player's current nutritional habits so that subtle changes can be made wherever necessary. Simply asking each team member to record everything she is eating for a short period of time—say, for 5 to 7 days—will provide the coach with a basic insight into individual dietary habits. Nevertheless, in cases where the coach does not feel able to give correct advice, assistance from appropriately qualified sports nutritionists should always be sought.

═Summary═

- Female players of team sports should be encouraged to consume a diet that contains a high proportion of carbohydrate. Recommendations for carbohydrate consumption depend on the individual's total energy intake. If she consumes *more than* 45 calories/kg of body weight per day, then a minimum of 55 percent of total energy intake should come from carbohydrate. If total energy intake is *less than* 45 calories/kg of body weight per day, then carbohydrate intake should be a minimum of 6 g/kg of body weight per day. (To determine body weight in kilograms, divide body weight in pounds by 2.2.) (See also Tables 5.1 and 5.2.)

- A high fluid intake should be maintained at all times.

- It is essential that female games players be encouraged to modify their energy intake to match their energy expenditure. Energy expenditure will of course change during the different phases of the season and also when activity levels are reduced for reasons such as injury or illness.

- Nutritional counseling should focus on the importance of carbohydrate to sustain training and playing, and should emphasize that, through the substitution of carbohydrate for fat, it is possible to increase carbohydrate intake without increasing total energy intake.

- Due to the time constraints placed upon women athletes who have to combine training and playing with other occupations, regular small meals with a high carbohydrate content are recommended.

5

- Vitamin supplementation should not be necessary if a person is consuming a diet of sufficient quantity, quality, and variety. However, particular attention should be given to calcium and iron intake in individuals who may be at risk of having a deficiency in these areas, thus emphasizing the fact that the dietary habits of all members within a team should be looked at on an individual basis.

- Nutritional counseling should include members of the athlete's family, who will need to assist in the provision of appropriate meals.

- Those advising women athletes on nutrition should be aware of the possible existence of, or the potential risk of inducing, disordered eating patterns.

- A correct nutritional strategy is vital if performance is to be sustained at a high level throughout the course of a season in which peaks in performance have to be achieved on a regular basis.

- In cases where the coach is concerned about the nutritional practices of any of his or her team members, assistance should always be sought from an appropriately qualified sports nutritionist.

Further Reading

J. Brewer, "Nutritional Aspects of Women's Soccer" (*Journal of Sports Sciences*, vol. 12, special issue, Summer 1994).

C. Economos, S. S. Bortz, M. E. Nelson, "Nutritional Practices of Elite Athletes: Practical Recommendations" (*Sports Medicine*, vol. 16, no. 6, 1993).

J. Nutter, "Seasonal Changes in Female Athletes' Diets" (*International Journal of Sports Nutrition*, vol. 1, 1991, pp. 395–407).

Acknowledgment

With grateful thanks to Sarah Smith for her assistance in the preparation of this chapter.

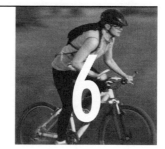

Body Fat and Weight Management

Professor N. C. Craig Sharp

Professor N. C. Craig Sharp, BVMS, MRCVS, Ph.D., FIBiol, FPEA, FBASAS, is Professor of Sports Science at Brunel University, Adjunct Professor of Sport Science at the University of Limerick, and former Director of Physiological Services at the British Olympic Medical Centre. His research interests include the physiology of elite athletes and the anatomical/physiological differences between sportsmen and -women.

Our bodies are made up of a wide variety of tissues, but for most of adult life the two tissues that cause major changes in body weight are muscle and fat. To a much lesser extent, alterations in blood and bone may also cause changes in weight; blood may increase by up to 1 kg (2.2 pounds) as one becomes aerobically fitter, and bone mass may increase with exercise (although bone mass tends to decrease starting at about age 35; by age 65 a bone loss of about 10 percent in men and 20 percent in women has occurred). For most women, however (not counting pregnancy), it is body fat, rather than muscle, that most influences body weight.

How Does Body Composition Change with Age?

At the age of 8, girls on average have approximately 18 percent body fat. During and following their adolescent growth spurt, they put on more fat than boys; girls' body fat increases to around 25 percent at the age of 17, and this may rise further in their early 20s. This fat increase at puberty, particularly around the hips and upper thighs, changes the center of gravity of a woman's body and also of the limb segments, and therefore may adversely affect performance in certain high-skill sports such as gymnastics, diving, trampolining, dance, and ice skating. Between the ages of 30 and 60, body fat percentage in the average sedentary woman increases steadily, at a rate of 1.5 to 2 percent per decade.

Does Body Composition Affect Sports Performance?

For *most* sports, a relatively low body fat percentage is advantageous for performance—excess fat tends to reduce speed, power, and stamina. However, this is not a straightforward linear relationship, since each individual has her own optimal fat level at which she will perform at her best. Moreover, attempts to reduce body fat levels through severe dieting, purging, or excessive exercise can result in depleted energy levels, depleted nutrient stores, and poor bone health, all of which adversely affect performance. Therefore, it is impossible to prescribe an ideal body fat percentage for any particular sport.

In women, the lowest body fat levels are found in middle- and long-distance runners, triathletes, dancers, and gymnasts (including rhythmic gymnasts), body builders, judoists (in the lower weight categories), and lightweight rowers. Body fat percentages may range from as low as 12 percent to around 20 percent. Women in team sports (such as hockey, basketball, soccer, volleyball, softball, lacrosse, etc.) and those in racket sports tend to range from 18 to 26 percent. Competitors in the athletic throwing events—especially in discus and shot—and rugby forwards usually vary between 25 and 32 percent. Perhaps the only serious women athletes with body fat percentages consistently above these levels are long-distance open-water swimmers, whose additional fat acts as a vital insulator and increases buoyancy, thus aiding the mechanics of the stroke (to very good effect, as many of the long-distance swimming records, including seven of the ten fastest English Channel swims, are held by women).

What Are the Different Types of Fat?

Our bodies contain two main types of fat: essential fat and storage fat. Essential fat is present as a constituent of the myelin, which insulates nerves, and as packing for vital organs (for example, the intraocular fat pad, which helps seat the eye in the orbit; fat around the kidneys, liver, and ovaries; some fat in the breast). Approximately 10 percent of the body weight of a slim woman consists of essential fat, compared to only 3 percent in an equivalent man. This sex-specific fat is needed for normal hormonal and reproductive functioning.

Storage fat, or adipose tissue, is primarily a fuel store supplying fuel for energy production in cells (including, of course, muscle cells). The whole body contains enough stored fat energy on which to stay alive for many weeks—or for 5 to 10 days of continual exercise (depending on the duration and the intensity of the activity). In addition, muscle has its own moderate supply of glycogen (the storage form of glucose), a fuel store that can last for about 3 hours of jogging. Fat is stored in fat cells or adipocytes. The average woman with 25 to 28 percent body fat has about 30 to 40 thousand million adipocytes, each containing about 45 micrograms of fat. With increasing fatness, the adipocytes may each gain up to twice this amount of fat.

The tissue known as "brown fat" is present in hibernating mammals, in babies and young children, and some persists in adults. Far from acting as an energy store, the function of this tissue is to metabolize fat at high rates, to generate heat, and thereby to stop such mammals from freezing to death. It has been postulated more generally to act as a "weight thermostat"—a "ponderostat"—to burn off excess calories, and so possibly to help regulate weight. However, its exact role in humans is still unclear.

How Important Is Storage Fat?

Fat is used for energy during all types of aerobic activities, including sitting, walking, and even sleeping. When we are exercising at low to moderate rates of exertion, as in walking, slow jogging, or slow swimming, a large proportion of the energy comes from fat. Indeed, at moderate levels of exertion such as these, fat is utilized directly from the fat depots via the blood to the muscles. It is only when the rate of exercise is increased, as in fast walking, running, or swimming, that the muscles start using more glycogen (and some glucose from the blood) and less fat. During anaerobic exercise (for example, sprinting and throwing), no fat is used at all.

Table 6.1: *Sex Differences in Percentage of Body Fat Between Men and Women in Their 20s*

Men	Women	Percent Fat
Thin		7
Average		12
Plump	Thin	18
Fat	Average	26
	Plump	31
	Fat	>36

6

The quantity of storage fat differs between men and women, with women generally having considerably more fat (see Table 6.1, which shows the approximate body fat percentages in various categories—from thin to fat). The difference in absolute quantity of fat between the sexes amounts to just enough to make a full-term baby (60,000–80,000 calories).

Incidentally, the extra fat mass is one of the main reasons why women's running events are slightly slower than men's—about 90 to 92 percent as fast. However, that same fat mass helps women to resist cold in swimming, sailing, mountain climbing, and polar expeditions, and therefore provides an advantage.

Can Low Body Fat Cause Amenorrhea?

There are a number of causes of amenorrhea or cessation of periods, including emotional or psychological stress, drug abuse, chronic illness, high volumes of strenuous training (as in endurance running, gymnastics, or rowing)—and marked weight loss or fat loss. Other factors being equal, lowering body weight or body fat below individual threshold levels will trigger amenorrhea, and subsequently increase the risk of premature bone loss, early osteoporosis, and possible stress fractures in sportswomen. Studies of runners have shown that those who were significantly lighter had higher rates of amenorrhea than their heavier counterparts with similar training and racing mileage. Also, in rowing, lightweight crews tend to have higher incidences of amenorrhea than heavyweight crews, although they are engaged in very similar training schedules and racing programs.

Weight and fat loss may act in two ways to produce or trigger this effect (even if it may only be the proverbial "last straw" in a complex process). First, a loss of weight and fat may act on the great integrating brain center, the hypothalamus, either directly or via higher nerve centers, causing it to lower its secretion of "pituitary releasing factors." These factors act on the main regulator of the body's hormones, the pituitary gland (sited just above the roof of the mouth), to depress its cyclic secretion of luteinizing and follicle-stimulating hormones. This in turn lowers the stimulus to the ovaries, causing them to secrete less of the sex hormones that periodically affect the uterus. Second, weight loss and—perhaps particularly—fat loss may directly influence the metabolism of the ovarian hormones that affect the uterus, reducing their effect. Thus, there may be a lower secretion of

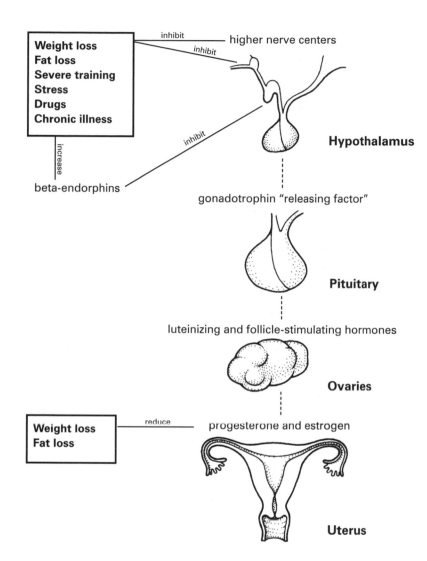

Weight loss
Fat loss
Severe training
Stress
Drugs
Chronic illness

inhibit ———— higher nerve centers
inhibit

increase

beta-endorphins

inhibit

Hypothalamus

gonadotrophin "releasing factor"

Pituitary

luteinizing and follicle-stimulating hormones

Ovaries

Weight loss
Fat loss

reduce ———— progesterone and estrogen

Uterus

Figure 6.1: *Possible association of irregular periods or amenorrhea with weight loss or fat loss. Loss of weight or of fat may, with various other factors, act through higher nerve centers in the brain, through the hypothalamus or via endorphins, to lower the secretion of "releasing factors" from the hypothalamus that normally stimulate the pituitary to produce luteinizing and follicle-stimulating hormones. Depression of these two pituitary hormones results in upset or failure of menstruation through cutting down the production of progesterone and estrogen, which prepare the uterus each month for pregnancy. Also, the loss of weight and fat may influence estrogen metabolism, which may also adversely affect the uterus. Note that weight loss and fat loss are implicated at two stages of the process.*

less effective hormones, and the uterus stops responding. These rather complex events are shown diagrammatically in Figure 6.1.

The percentage of body fat below which amenorrhea develops varies markedly from one person to the next. It can be anywhere between 15 and 20 percent. Thus, weight loss or a loss of fat to very low percentages may trigger amenorrhea. Similarly, an increase of weight or fat usually induces a revival of normal periods. For more information on this topic, refer to Chapter 4.

How Can Body Fat Be Measured?

There are numerous methods of varying sophistication for measuring body fat, but determining the thickness of the skin at specific sites with skinfold calipers is the simplest and by far the most widely used method of gaining a useful estimate. The skin is itself a fat depot, and it correlates fairly well with the other fat depots in the body. Appearances can be very deceptive; some slim-looking women have surprisingly high body fat, while some plumper-looking women can be surprisingly muscular underneath and carry less fat than one might think. The main fat depots in women are typically (though not always) the thighs, hips, back of the arms, and bust, while in men the abdomen (the beer belly) is usually the principal site of fat storage.

There are two other, less direct methods of assessing body fat status: the body mass index and the waist/hip ratio.[2]

Body Mass Index

The body mass index (BMI) is calculated as follows: (1) weigh yourself in kilograms (weight in pounds divided by 2.2); (2) measure your height in meters (height in inches times 0.025); (3) square your height in meters; (4) divide your weight in kilograms (step 1) by your squared height (step 3).

Example:

(1) 140 pounds divided by 2.2 = 63.64 kg

(2) 65 inches times 0.025 = 1.625 meters

(3) 1.625 times 1.625 = 2.641

(4) 63.64 kg divided by 2.641 = 24.1

Table 6.2: *Male and Female Body Mass Index Categories (not body fat percentages)*

Male	Body Mass Index	Distribution in the UK (% of national survey)
Underweight	20 or less	4%
Acceptable	20.1–25	47%
Overweight	25.1–30	41%
Obese	Over 30	8%
Female	**Body Mass Index**	**Distribution in the UK (% of national survey)**
Underweight	18.6 or less	2%
Acceptable	18.7–23.8	42%
Overweight	23.9–28.5	37%
Obese	Over 28.5	19%

(Source: Royal Society of Physicians (UK))

The Royal College of Physicians in the UK has prepared a table of BMI values, reproduced here as Table 6.2.

The BMI tends to reflect body fat increases: your weight changes, but your height stays relatively constant. So, the lower one's weight becomes, the lower the BMI. The problem with BMI for athletes is that it uses a single value for simple body mass, and no account is taken of whether this weight contains a lot of muscle or a lot of fat. Also, athletes and women on exercise programs may lose fat and put on muscle and other tissues, so their weight may stay the same (or even increase slightly) although their body composition may have changed decidedly for the better (as shown in Figure 6.2). However, the BMI is a useful guide in health terms for most women—and may prompt some into a health-related activity program.

The usual threshold for defining overweight in women (and men) is a BMI of between 25 to 30, and for *obesity* a BMI of over 30. On this scale, nearly 53 percent of men and 44 percent of women are in the overweight or obese category. However, the Royal Society of Physicians proposed a different (harder) scale for women (shown in Table 6.2) whereby well over 50 percent of women would be classified as overweight or above. Nevertheless, in health terms—according to major surveys correlating death risk and BMI—BMIs of between 23 and 29 for women appear to be the healthiest. It is probably worse to be much below 21 than it is to be as far above 31.

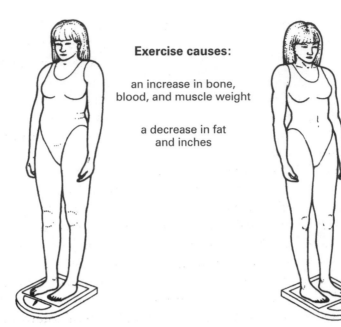

Exercise causes:

an increase in bone,
blood, and muscle weight

a decrease in fat
and inches

Start of exercise program
125 lbs.

Two months later
125 lbs.

Figure 6.2: Body Weight vs. Body Composition. Body weight may not change much in the early stages of an exercise program, although body composition may well change appreciably.

In the 1990s, Australian researchers strongly challenged the focus of attention given to overweight women, stating, "men and boys are at a far higher risk of the medical complications of obesity than women and girls." Bill Tuxworth, field director of the National Fitness Survey, noted the paradox that "men—who have most to fear from obesity—are under little pressure to control their weight, while women and girls, for most of whom obesity is a minor health problem, develop excessive weight preoccupations." In Australia, well over 90 percent of all persons who are under treatment for obesity are female, which led top researcher Dr. Stunkard to deplore "the strong social pressures towards thinness, which are exerted on women as early as 10 years of age." There is a strong concern that a literal interpretation of even some of the health promotion material could induce some women into over-thinness. This is dealt with in more detail in Chapter 8.

If women in the upper half of the 20 to 30 BMI range find that they have suddenly put on weight over the past few months—for example, through giving up smoking, being injured, or changing jobs (*not* through pregnancy!)—then they should seek professional help from a qualified nutritionist early on to halt the increase in body fat by an achievable, realistic combination of exercise and diet.

Waist/Hip Ratio

The other method of measuring body composition is the waist/hip ratio, which is simply the measurement of the waist in inches or centimeters divided by that of the hips. For women (because of their proportionately larger pelvic hip bones), the ratio should be at or below 0.8. For men, it should be less than 1.0. For example, a woman with a waist measurement of 26″ (66 cm) and hips of 36″ (91.4 cm) has a waist/hip ratio of 26 ÷ 36 = 0.72. In metric terms the ratio would be the same (66 ÷ 91.4 = 0.72).

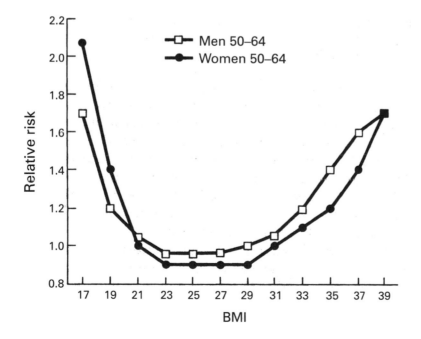

Figure 6.3: *Relative Risk of Death According to Body Mass Index*

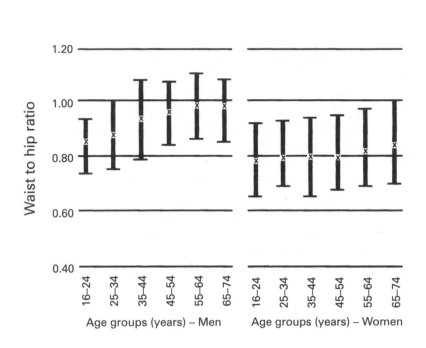

Figure 6.4: *Waist/Hip Ratio of Men and Women by Age (from ADNFS). Each bar indicates the range of the majority in each age group.*

The waist/hip ratio is also an important health measure, although more in men than in women. Excess fat in the abdomen is considered to be more harmful than excess fat elsewhere, due to its greater correlation with heart attacks. A man with a waist of 46" (117 cm) and hips of 42" (107 cm), a ratio of 46 ÷ 42 = 1.1, has double the chance of having a heart attack than if he had a W/H ratio of below 1.0. Women's chances of a heart attack increase to some extent if this ratio rises above 0.8, although it should be emphasized that this correlation is not nearly as clear-cut as that of men. Again, there is a greater medical risk in obese men than in women. In both sexes, the W/H ratio will fall as body fat is lost. Figure 6.4 shows the W/H ratio results from the Allied Dunbar National Fitness Survey, with the range found in each age group.

Finally, simple measurements with a tape measure can be made of the circumference of the upper arms, thighs, calves, bust, waist, and hip. These can be monitored: loss of circumference will usually denote a loss of fat (and vice-versa). Indeed, this is one of the best measures of all!

How Can I Reduce Body Fat?

The average woman eats about 20 tons (over 20,000 kg) of food between the ages of 25 and 65, yet she only gains 11 kg (24 pounds) in that time. In other words, even without any conscious attempt at weight control, we are regulating our weight to less than a single gram per day (less than $\frac{1}{28}$ of an ounce). So, a very powerful regulator is at work. And it does not take much to tilt the balance one way or the other.

The important point to realize is that the body obeys the laws of thermodynamics. It neither creates nor destroys energy. Fat is an energy store. Therefore, fat accumulates if more food energy is ingested than physical and muscular energy are expended. However, if more physical and muscular energy are expended than food energy ingested, then fat diminishes.

Therefore, to lose fat, one either has to eat less while maintaining the same energy output, or to exercise more while maintaining the same energy intake. In practice, it is best to do a bit of both—to expend more calories by increasing physical exercise, and to eat less energy. Exercise also has a degree of "afterburner" effect, due to the exercise triggering an adrenaline release which may maintain a higher rate of metabolism for an hour or two after the effort—or even more following longer periods of vigorous exercise.

If a person eats 100 calories fewer each day (equivalent to two small crackers) and expends an extra 100 calories (equivalent to 20 to 30 minutes of moderate walking), then the calorie deficit would amount to the equivalent of 8.1 kg (18 pounds) of fat a year. And this is the way to think about fat loss—a gradual reduction in the long term (up to a year). Severe calorie restriction can depress the metabolic rate by up to 30 percent, and by as much as 45 percent on a very low calorie diet: the body switches into "starvation mode" and becomes much more economical, hence much less food is needed. Thus, what started out as a diet may turn into a relative calorie excess! Also, crash diets tend initially to empty the muscle reserves of two or three kg (4.4–6.6 pounds) of glycogen. And since each kilogram (2.2 pounds) of glycogen stores three kg (6.6 pounds) of water with it, the "weight loss" on a crash diet can be very dramatic indeed for the first few days, due simply to glycogen and water depletion. Weight will be regained rapidly once carbohydrate intake is increased.

Diet or Exercise?

Evidence is accumulating to support the suggestion that exercise may be more effective than dieting in the maintenance of a desirable body composition. In one experiment, for example, three groups of people were put on a weight-loss program representing a daily deficit of 500 calories. In one group this was reached solely by eating 500 fewer calories; in the second group by 250 calories fewer in terms of food and by 250 calories more in terms of exercise; and in the third group solely by using 500 calories more per day through exercise. The individuals in all three groups each lost 5 kg (11 pounds) over 16 weeks: in the first group, 1.1 kg (2.5 pounds) of this loss was muscle; the second group gained 1 kg (2.2 pounds) of muscle and lost 6 kg (13 pounds) of fat; while the third group gained 2.2 kg (4.8 pounds) of muscle and lost 7 kg (15 pounds) of fat.

In other words, the diet-only group lost muscle and fat, the exercise-and-diet group gained some muscle and lost more fat, while the exercise-only group gained quite a lot of muscle and lost the most fat.

This illustrates the point that dieting on its own is unhealthy in that muscle is lost as well as fat—which is not the object in dieting. For most people, exercising to the equivalent of 500 calories a day is too much: it equals 35 minutes of squash or other equally vigorous activity, or 60 to 90 minutes of hard cycling, aerobics, or similar exercise; 200 calories per day is a more realistic target. Also, it should be noted that the energy costs of activities vary according to body weight and conditions (see Tables 6.3 and 6.4, which give examples for walking).

Table 6.3: The energy expenditure in calories per minute of people of different body weights walking at different speeds on level ground

Mph	km/h	36 kg 80 lbs.	45 kg 100 lbs.	54 kg 120 lbs.	64 kg 140 lbs.	73 kg 160 lbs.	82 kg 180 lbs.	91 kg 200 lbs.
2	3.2	1.9	2.2	2.6	2.9	3.2	3.5	3.8
2½	4.0	2.3	2.7	3.1	3.5	3.8	4.2	4.5
3	4.8	2.7	3.1	3.6	4.0	4.4	4.8	5.3
3½	5.6	3.1	3.6	4.2	4.6	5.0	5.4	6.1
4	6.4	3.5	4.1	4.7	5.2	5.8	6.4	7.0

Table 6.4: Energy costs of walking on different surfaces vary by these approximate correction factors

Terrain	Correction factor
Road	1.0
Grass	1.1
Stubble field	1.2
Plowed field	1.4
Firm snow	1.6
Loose sand	1.8
On level ground against 40 mph wind	Over 3.0

What Is the Difference Between Fat Loss and Weight Loss?

A combination of modest diet and modest exercise is important. Nevertheless, many people are disappointed during the early months of a program that includes exercise because they do not lose weight more quickly—even though they may lose *fat*. A program that includes exercise will result in some increase in muscle mass (not bulk), including a slightly larger glycogen store in the muscle, the blood volume will beneficially increase, and there will be some increase in tendon and bone (see Figure 6.2). So loss of *fat* is not always accompanied by an equivalent loss in *weight*.

A minor spin-off of an exercise program is that in people who are very sedentary, appetite tends to "free-wheel," whereas even modest regular exercise tends to lock appetite more into need. So when very sedentary people start a modest exercise program, they often find that they feel like eating less, because they start to regain their natural appetite cues.

Body fat estimation, by skinfold measurement, for example, should confirm the drop in fat, even though the weight may not have changed much. Limb, waist, and hip circumference measures should confirm changes in contour also, and back, thighs, and arms may feel agreeably firmer to the touch. As the program goes on through the months, the increase in lean body mass will stabilize and weight will gradually fall as fat is lost.

What Is the Best Form of Exercise?

In exercising for fat loss, the critical factor is the total calories used, not the intensity of the effort. For example, squash may use 15 calories per minute, so 30 minutes = 450 calories; whereas a game of golf may use only 5 calories per minute but take 3 hours, 180 minutes x 5 = 900 calories. So, for *fat-losing* purposes, a game of golf is twice as good as a game of squash (although the vigorous effort involved in an intense game of squash will promote a better "afterburner" effect).

Regular exercise has many other health and fitness benefits. It strengthens the heart, lowers blood pressure, improves blood profile of fats and cholesterol, improves lung capacity, helps to prevent diabetes, improves the health of the immune system, and strengthens joints. In terms of lifestyle-related fitness, it improves stamina, strength, and flexibility and maintains good bone health. Another major benefit of exercise is that it improves your mood and has many other psychological benefits (related to changes in brain chemistry)—indeed, it is used increasingly as a nondrug treatment of depression.

For exercise to benefit your bones—to help slow the rate of osteoporosis or the thinning of bone that occurs with aging—the main thing is that the exercise be weight bearing. This gives the bone a proper stimulus. (See Chapter 4 for further discussion of this topic.) Thus, brisk walking, jogging, tennis, badminton, squash, aerobics, and country and disco dance are much better—for bones—than swimming and cycling.

It is particularly important to stress that fat loss not be overdone, or overemphasized—especially in women in the 15-to-25-year-old age group, in whom the risk of anorexia is greatest. It is largely fat which gives women an "aesthetic shape," however that may be defined. Above a certain age, a slightly full figure may be pleasingly accompanied by a less drawn face; and for people over 30, a reasonable amount of fat—25 to 30 percent in women and 15 to 20 percent in men—is "programmed" to be there. It is perfectly possible to be very fit and healthy, yet not be overly thin. The skeletally based fashion industry pays no attention to health needs in its depictions of women. Clothes shops should perhaps stop using mannequins that, if they were real women, would often be too thin to menstruate!

═Practical Points ═

- Women who participate in regular exercise or play sports generally have lower body fat levels (12 to 26 percent) than nonactive women, with the lowest percentages (12 to 20 percent) found in middle- and long-distance runners, triathletes, gymnasts, and those competing in weight-category sports.

- Total body fat comprises essential fat (approximately 10 percent in women) and storage fat (approximately 16 percent in average women). Sex-specific essential fat is necessary for normal hormonal and menstrual functions in women.

- Weight and fat loss to very low levels (usually less than 15 to 20 percent body fat) may trigger amenorrhea and increase the risk of bone loss and stress fractures.

- Body mass index (BMI) and waist/hip (W/H) ratio are useful health measures for most women. Skinfold-thickness measurements are a simple and relatively accurate, practical method for estimating body fat in exercising women.

- Body fat reduction should be gradual (1–2 pounds per week or less) and achieved by a combination of diet and increased aerobic exercise.

- A fat-burning exercise program should take account of the total calories used as well as the intensity.

- A certain amount of body fat is functionally vital and aesthetically desirable; less is not necessarily better for performance or health.

- Decide on a realistic body composition goal that will not compromise your health or training ability. Get professional guidance.

- Use a combination of skinfold thickness measurements and circumference measurements to monitor changes in body composition; and set a suitable and realistic time frame for weight loss and fat loss.

- Amenorrhea or menstrual irregularities may be reversed by gradual weight gain, reducing training load, or reducing psychological stress—or a combination of all three. If in doubt, consult a sports physician or a sports nutritionist.

Notes

1. Free radicals are atoms or molecules generated during normal energy production which contain an unpaired electron. In large numbers they are capable of damaging cell membranes and DNA, and of oxidizing blood cholesterol; they are thought to be responsible for initiating certain cancers and heart disease.

2. For detailed tables by age for both BMI and waist/hip ratio, see appendix A of the *Allied Dunbar National Fitness Survey*, published in 1992 by the Sports Council (UK).

Further Reading

Allied Dunbar National Fitness Survey (Sports Council and Health Education Authority [UK], 1992).

W. McArdle, F. Katch, V. Katch, *Exercise Physiology, Energy, Nutrition and Human Performance* (Lea and Febiger, 1991, 3d ed.).

R. Passmore, J. Durnin, *Energy, Work and Leisure* (Heinemann, 1967).

"Obesity Report" (Royal College of Physicians [UK], *Journal of the Royal College of Physicians*, vol. 17, no. 50, 1983, p. 65).

N. C. C. Sharp, *Fully Fit Through Walking* (Patrick Stephens, 1988).

A. J. Stunkard, "Obesity: Risk Factors, Consequences and Control" (*Medical Journal of Australia*, vol. 148, 1988, pp. 521–28).

W. Tuxworth, "What Should Public Health Policy Be Towards 'Overweight'?" (British Nutrition Foundation, *Nutrition Bulletin*, vol. 19, 1994, pp. 24–26).

H. Waaler, "Weight and Mortality: The Norwegian Experience" (*Acta Medica, Scandinavia*, 215, supplement 679, 1984, pp. 1–56).

Acknowledgements

I wish to express very grateful thanks to Bill Tuxworth, field director of the Allied Dunbar National Fitness Survey, for his generosity in helping with this contribution and for his splendid scientific comradeship over the past 25 years, and to John Durnin for firing my interest in body composition with his stimulating work and discussions even longer ago.

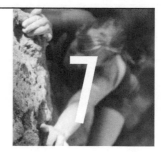

7

Practical Weight-Loss Strategies

Anita Bean, B.Sc.

Does Excess Body Fat Affect Performance?

Having a particular body fat percentage for a particular sport is regarded by many women as an increasingly important issue.

Carrying excess body fat is a distinct disadvantage for most sports and fitness activities. It can adversely affect your performance, reducing your power, speed, and endurance. For example, in endurance sports such as long-distance running, excess fat tends to reduce running speed and induce earlier fatigue. It has been estimated that a 5 percent decrease in body fat in a 160-pound runner could knock 6 minutes off a marathon time. In explosive and power sports such as sprinting, long jump, or volleyball, excess fat tends to reduce mechanical efficiency and therefore reduce performance.

Can You Go Too Low?

Obviously, there is a desirable range of body fat percentages for a particular sport or fitness activity; the relationship between performance and body fat is certainly not a linear one. However, a major problem is that many exercising women become tempted to take this link between body fat/weight and performance to the extreme in the misguided belief that the lower their body fat the better.

As fat percentage decreases below a certain level, this can have an adverse effect on performance. Long-term food restriction inevitably leads to depleted glycogen stores, incomplete recovery, slower tissue repair and formation, and reduced nutrient intake. The ultimate results are chronic fatigue, increased susceptibility to infections, reduced performance, over-training syndrome ("burnout"), increased risk of iron deficiency anemia, premature bone loss, and greater risk of injury.

The other major problem is the development of disordered eating patterns or subclinical and clinical eating disorders, such as anorexia nervosa and bulimia nervosa. American studies suggest that around 60 percent of normal-weight young women have some form of disordered eating. One particular study of gymnasts carried out at the University of North Texas found that only 22 percent could be classified as having normal eating habits. Sixty-one percent had a subclinical eating disorder, and 16 percent had bulimia nervosa. Researchers agree that such eating behavior is common among other groups of female athletes and exercisers, particularly in individuals who tend to have a low self-esteem. This subject of body image and dieting is dealt with in more detail in Chapter 8.

What Is a Desirable Percentage of Body Fat?

It is impossible to define an exact value for any particular sport. Certainly a range is acceptable, and this will depend on the individual woman. It is unlikely that any two people will have exactly the same "optimal" level of body fat. For example, one swimmer may perform at her best with 16 percent fat, while her teammate may perform equally well with 18 percent.

For women, 18–25 percent is considered desirable from a health point of view, although for competitive athletes the percentage is likely to be lower. One study has suggested 13–18 percent for women as optimal for performance in most sports requiring a lean physique. However, bear in mind that this range is not necessarily optimal for health.

Should We Count Calories?

Counting calories may become a thing of the past. A growing amount of research suggests that calories from carbohydrate, fat, or protein are handled in quite different ways in the body and this, in turn, has an important bearing on body-fat levels. Rather than simply considering overall energy balance (calories in versus calories out), scientists are now looking at the separate balance equations of each macronutrient (the macronutrients are nutrients that contain calories: protein, fat, and carbohydrate). In other words, carbohydrate intake versus carbohydrate oxidation or storage; fat intake versus fat oxidation or storage; and so on.

The hypothesis that fat is more fattening calorie for calorie than carbohydrate is supported by a number of well-controlled studies. In a study of prisoners in Vermont, it was found that lean men gained weight more readily when overfed a high-fat diet than when overfed a mixed diet of carbohydrate and fat. In another recent study, men were fed 150 percent of their calorie requirements for two 14-day periods. In one period the excess calories came from fat; in the other the excess calories came from carbohydrate. Overfeeding fat caused much greater deposition of body fat than overfeeding carbohydrate. What's more, this effect was magnified in the men who were already obese.

Can Alcohol Increase Body Fat?

Alcohol cannot be stored in the body since it is toxic. Therefore, all alcohol ingested is broken down and ultimately converted into energy. While this is happening, it suppresses the oxidation of fat. So, indirectly, alcohol may affect body fat levels by channeling fat into fat storage.

Can Carbohydrate Increase Body Fat?

Carbohydrate consumed in excess of the body's immediate needs can be stored in the muscles as glycogen. However, stores are relatively small (approximately 400 g) and tightly controlled. Studies show that when carbohydrate is overeaten, it actually increases carbohydrate oxidation. In other words, some of the excess carbohydrate is merely burned off and effectively wasted as heat. As much as one-quarter of the calories from carbohydrate are converted into excess heat, and the rest is preferentially converted into glycogen.

Does Dietary Fat Increase Body Fat?

In sharp contrast to the other nutrients, stores of fat are extremely large (enough for the average person to jog 800 miles!). Any fat eaten that is not immediately required for energy or metabolism is stored in adipose (fat) tissue. Overeating fat does not increase fat oxidation, nor does it affect appetite. Fat oxidation is only increased when total energy demands exceed total energy intake or during aerobic exercise.

Leading researchers into obesity have proposed another physiological theory to explain why fat is easily overconsumed. Even in the short term, they say, it is not as satiating as other nutrients. Fat is not metabolized as rapidly after meals as carbohydrate or protein. While carbohydrate produces a rise in blood glucose, fat often depresses blood glucose, which means carbohydrate produces more rapid satiety than fat.

What Is the Secret of Appetite Control?

Appetite is tightly controlled by the relative amounts of carbohydrate, fat, and protein we eat. Glycogen plays the biggest role in regulating hunger and appetite and therefore in achieving long-term weight management.

Fluctuations in our glycogen stores are detected by our appetite control centers and translated into feelings of hunger. So, when glycogen stores are low we experience an increased appetite and have a desire to eat more. When glycogen stores are full, our appetite is reduced and we eat less. Therefore, carbohydrate balance is achieved partly through increased oxidation and partly through appetite control.

So How Can Carbohydrates Help Weight Loss?

A diet high in complex carbohydrates and low in fat means it is almost impossible to overeat and gain weight. Carbohydrates have a satiating effect on our appetite while fat has practically no appetite-dampening effect at all. We could happily overeat high-fat foods for days on end without any decrease in our appetite. But with high-carbohydrate foods, we would feel full much more quickly.

A recent study carried out at the Dunn Clinical Nutrition Center (Cambridge, England) shows that volunteers allowed unlimited access to a low-fat (20 percent calories from fat), high-carbohydrate diet for 7 days unwittingly lost body fat. However, when they were fed a medium-fat diet (40 percent of calories from fat) or a high-fat diet (60 percent of calories from fat) *which looked exactly the same*, they overate and gained up to 0.9 kg body fat. The volunteers said they did not notice any difference in taste between the low-fat and high-fat diets and that their appetites were fully satisfied on both.

A series of recent experiments carried out at the Human Appetite Research Unit at Leeds University found that when volunteers were given a high-carbohydrate breakfast, then allowed an unlimited amount of a snack meal 1½ hours later, they voluntarily ate fewer calories compared with when they ate a higher-fat breakfast. It was concluded that adding extra fat to the breakfast had no effect on appetite control for the rest of the day. On the other hand, adding extra carbohydrate to the breakfast reduced hunger for longer—volunteers had less desire to eat snacks later on and were unlikely to overeat during the day.

What Are the Dangers of Strict Dieting?

The main problem with cutting your calories too severely is that you will not be getting enough food to maintain your essential tissues (organs, muscles, bones, etc.) and all your essential body processes (breathing, digestion, blood circulation, kidney function, etc). The number of calories your body uses at rest is described as its resting metabolic rate (RMR). For most women the RMR is between 1,200 and 1,500 calories per day. The heavier you are and the more muscular you are, the higher your metabolic rate. So a larger person uses up more calories than a small person. An athlete uses up more calories than a sedentary person of the same weight.

If you eat less than your RMR, you will encourage your body to break down protein, which will come from muscle tissue and possibly from organ tissue too. So you lose not only fat but also valuable lean tissue.

Remember that you use extra calories whenever you move about, whether that's walking, shopping, or exercising. So your total calorie output will be quite a bit higher than your RMR. The higher your caloric intake the greater chance you have of getting enough vitamins, minerals, and protein, because you are eating more food. Although it is possible to get enough vitamins and minerals from 1,000 calories worth of food, in practice this is quite hard to achieve. For a start, you'd have to eat a very wide variety of foods and include plenty of fresh fruit and vegetables. Many exercisers with a busy lifestyle tend to rely on high-fat snacks, calorie-counted, readymade meals, and other convenience foods, which might be low in certain vitamins. It is all too easy to miss out on valuable nutrients like calcium, iron, vitamin E, and vitamin A.

How Can I Reduce Body Fat?

The healthiest and most effective way to lose body fat is through a combination of diet and exercise. Here is a simple eight-point plan to help you reduce your body-fat level safely and healthily without compromising performance.

1. Goal Setting

Decide on a *realistic* goal or, better still, a series of short-term goals that can definitely be achieved. Discuss this with a sports nutritionist, your coach, or a professional instructor, taking into account your own body type, shape, and present training program. Progress is best monitored by a combination of skinfold thickness measurements and circumference measurements at key sites, rather than by weighing on the scales.

2. Estimate Your Present Calorie Intake

Everyone's calorie requirements are different, depending on body weight, activity level, body composition, and individual metabolism. Start with your current calorie intake by writing an accurate food diary for at least three days. Be sure to record every bite you eat, and be accurate about the portions. Bear in mind that 1 pound of fat provides 3,500 calories. So you need to create a deficit of 3,500 calories over a 1-week period to lose 1 pound of fat. That is equivalent to 500 calories per day and may be done by eating less and exercising more.

Be patient! Do not attempt to lose more than 1 or 2 pounds a week—otherwise your body will break down excessive muscle and organ tissue. So, if you normally eat 2,500 calories a day, reduce to 2,000 calories.

3. Do Not Eat Less Than Your RMR

For most women, the RMR is 1,200–1,500 calories a day—the minimum intake required to maintain lean body mass. Going lower than this will encourage your body to break down protein and glycogen. To get a rough idea of your own RMR, simply multiply your weight in pounds by 10. For example, if you weigh 126 pounds, then your RMR is roughly 1,260 calories. Therefore, you would need a minimum of 1,260 calories to simply survive (at rest) for 1 day.

4. Keep Carbohydrate Intake High

Aim to get at least 60 percent of your calories from carbohydrates. Many people cut down on high-carbohydrate foods in the mistaken belief that this will help them lose weight. The problem lies not with carbohydrates but with fat! Carbohydrates are *not* "fattening" (they contain less than half the calories of fats) and are essential for ensuring maximum fuel stores for exercise. Remember, a high-carbohydrate, low-fat diet makes it almost impossible to overeat and gain body fat!

The good-carbohydrate guide

- All types of bread (including multigrain, rye, soda, cracked wheat, rolls, bagels; be wary of eating muffins—many contain excessive amounts of fat)

- Breakfast cereals

- Dishes based on pasta, rice, oats, couscous, barley, millet

- Baked, boiled, and mashed potatoes or sweet potatoes

- Beans, lentils, peas

- Starchy vegetables such as parsnips, yams, corn, plantains

- Fresh, dried, and canned fruit

---

5. Cut Down—But Not Out—Fat!

Since fat is the most concentrated source of calories (9 calories/g, compared with carbohydrate and protein at 4 calories/g each), reduce your intake of high-fat foods. However, do not aim to eliminate fat altogether, because a certain amount is necessary in order to obtain the essential fatty acids and help to absorb and utilize the fat-soluble vitamins. A very low fat diet, if followed for a long period of time, may lead to hormonal imbalances, lower vitamin status, dry skin, and other health problems. It will also mean a very low intake of important antioxidant nutrients such as vitamin

E (which can help reduce free-radical damage, heart disease risk, and the risk of certain cancers, and may slow down the aging process). You should include a small amount of fat- or oil-containing foods in your daily diet, preferably from vegetable sources, e.g., olive oil, sunflower oil, nuts, peanut butter, seeds.

Cut down on:

- Butter, margarine, and other spreading fats
- Deep-fried foods, such as French fries
- Fatty meats and meat products, e.g., beef burgers, sausages, bacon
- Pastries
- Cakes, cookies, desserts
- Chocolate and other candy
- Chips and similar snacks

Choose instead:

- Very low fat spread, peanut butter, tahini
- Grilled/microwaved/boiled/baked/stir-fried foods
- Well-trimmed, lean cuts of meat
- Chicken and turkey (skinned, white meat)
- Tuna packed in water
- Pasta and rice dishes without oily or creamy sauces
- Low-fat yogurt
- Rice pudding, Fig Newtons, crackers
- Rice cakes, oat cakes

6. *Eat Frequent and Regular Snacks/Meals*

Small, regular meals and snacks help keep your blood sugar and insulin levels more stable, avoiding fluctuations in your energy levels. Research shows that this pattern of eating helps to reduce blood cholesterol levels. Equally important, your body is then assured of a more steady supply of nutrients to replenish glycogen stores, speed up recovery between workouts, and maximize your body's response to exercise (e.g., muscle tissue repair, strengthening, toning).

The healthy-snack guide

- Sandwiches, rolls, pita bread, bagels with low-fat fillings (banana, cottage cheese, tuna, chicken, salad, hummus spread)

- Low fat muffins, fruit buns, scones

- Oat cakes and rice cakes with low-fat toppings (banana, fruit spread)

- Toast with honey/fruit spread/baked beans

- Fresh fruit (bananas, apples, pears, grapes)

- Dried fruit (raisins, apricots, dates, apples)

- Dried fruit bars, cereal bars

- Homemade shakes made with low-fat milk, bananas, and yogurt

- Baked potatoes with low-fat toppings (cottage cheese, baked beans, salsa)

- Breakfast cereals with low-fat milk

7. Eat Breakfast

Skipping breakfast will not help you lose weight. U.S. studies have clearly shown that breakfast skippers are more likely to be overweight than people who regularly eat breakfast. The problem with missing out on this important meal is that it increases your hunger later on, making you more likely to overeat at mealtimes or nibble on high-calorie snacks. Consciously denying your hunger in the morning can also upset your body's natural appetite cues so you may lose your normal sensation and control of hunger and fullness. Again, this can cause you to overeat at mealtimes.

Eating breakfast will boost your blood-sugar levels and therefore your energy levels, stimulate your metabolism, and give you a significant proportion of your daily intake of vitamins, minerals, fiber, and carbohydrate. It is not essential that you eat breakfast immediately after getting up if you don't feel hungry, but do make a point of eating in the early part of the morning.

The good-breakfast guide

- Hot cereal (oatmeal, cream of wheat) made with skim or low-fat milk and served with fruit

- Whole-grain cereal such as bran or wheat flakes, shredded wheat, crunchy oat-based cereals (granola) and muesli, plus skim or low-fat milk

- Bagels and muffins with honey, plus fresh fruit

- Whole-meal toast with fruit spread, honey, peanut butter, marmalade, or jam

- Fresh fruit and dried fruit with low-fat yogurt (and nuts/seeds if you wish)

- Poached, boiled, or scrambled egg on whole-grain toast

8. Avoid Overeating in the Evening

If you exercise in the evening, aim to consume most of your food during the daytime. Have a substantial breakfast and lunch and include regular snacks in between. After exercise, have a high-carbohydrate snack or meal (for example, baked potato with a low-fat topping), enough to start refueling your glycogen reserves, but not so much that you feel bloated and overfull.

Try to leave at least a couple of hours after your main evening meal before going to sleep. Going to bed on a full stomach can make you feel uncomfortable and restless. If you eat a large meal before bedtime, most of the energy (calories) in the food will have to be stored rather than used for immediate energy needs. Some will be converted into glycogen (the body's carbohydrate store), but quite a lot may be converted into body fat.

A Note on Detoxification Diets

So-called detoxification diets are an extreme form of dieting. Theoretically, they claim to eliminate toxins (poisons) from the body and to "cleanse" the system by placing a short-term and drastic restriction on the range of foods you are allowed to eat. Most comprise just a few types of food, such as fruits and vegetables or fruit/vegetable juices.

There is no scientific proof that this type of dieting works, despite its fashionable image; nor is it recommended by scientifically trained doctors or nutritionists. You will probably lose weight in the short term (mostly glycogen and water) since you end up eating fewer calories, but such diets are neither a healthy nor a lasting solution to a weight problem. They should certainly not be followed for any period of time, as they can cause nutritional imbalances in the body. You should aim for a long-term, balanced, healthy eating program rather than a short-term quick fix. *Avoid any diet that goes to extremes.*

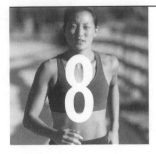

Body Image and Eating Disorders

Anita Bean, B.Sc.

Most women in the Western world have a distorted body image, perceiving themselves to be fatter than they really are. Many consequently spend a lifetime in pursuit of a leaner, lighter body. While some resort to the drastic measure of cosmetic surgery, most choose to focus on exercise and food intake. However, diet and exercise combined with a distorted body image can lead to an obsessive preoccupation with weight and calories, and eventually to disordered eating.

Women in the fitness or sports environment may be thought to harbor a more relaxed and positive attitude toward body image. It seems, however, that even in this context of heightened physical awareness, weight and aesthetics are becoming inextricably entwined with health, fitness, and performance.

This chapter examines the influences on body image of women in general and how they respond to the pressure to be thin, and also explores to what extent these attitudes are reflected in the exercise environment.

The Changing Shape of the Ideal Female Form

Throughout the ages, the conception of the ideal female shape has changed dramatically according to the trends of contemporary fashion. From the Rubenesque curves of the fifteenth century to the wasp waists and emphasized posteriors of the seventeenth and nineteenth centuries, women have resorted to corsets, bustles, and boning to conform to the fashionable shape. The fashion dictates of the twentieth century have, however, proven the most demanding. Women taped down their bosoms for the flapper girl flatness of the 1920s, mimicked Marilyn Monroe's curves in the 1950s, starved themselves for '60s-style androgyny, and exercised for muscles in the fitness boom of the 1970s and '80s. Currently, the media's choice of the ideal shape for the woman of the new millennium is personified by models such as Kate Moss, whose waiflike proportions (size 2 or 4 and 5'7" tall) promote a body shape unattainable by the majority of women.

How the changing female form has been artificially dictated by fashion trends rather than by nature is clearly shown in a study reported in the *British Medical Journal*, in which two Finnish doctors compare the measurements of shop-window mannequins with those of the average woman. They found that the mannequins' hips were 6" smaller and their thighs 4" thinner. Since World War II mannequins' proportions have shrunk dramatically by 4" around the hips and 2" around the thighs. A woman with a mannequin's body-fat ratio would in fact be malnourished, weak, amenorrheic, and even infertile, but in the fashion world a healthy body shape is all too frequently sacrificed for aesthetics.

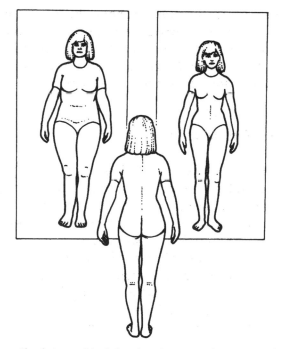

Figure 8.1: The term "body image" is defined as the internal picture we have of our bodies.

8

Why Should Women Be Thin?

In the media, thinness often symbolizes success, happiness, and self-control, while fat is equated with ugliness, lack of discipline, and misery. In reality, many slim women may diet and starve, sacrificing happiness for aesthetic gain. Who is behind this media propaganda? One feminist theory is that gay fashion designers select models whose form resembles that of teenage boys. Another is that women, increasingly competing with men on a business and social level, are pressured to be thin by a male "conspiracy" that seeks to suppress their encroachment on a male-dominated world: by literally taking up less space, women become less worthy of attention. Also, if a woman's focus is diverted to a preoccupation with her appearance, her self-confidence will be challenged and her threat lessened.

Women themselves are partly to blame for the obsession with thinness. Camille Paglia, feminist and controversial author of books on women's roles and personae, believes women compete with each other to be thin, often using this as a status symbol. That competition can clearly be seen in all-female environments such as girls' schools, where eating disorders can become endemic due to peer-group pressure.

Do Men Suffer Eating Disorders?

For men, the pressure to be thin is less intense, and the media more generous in its choice of the ideal shape. Indeed, largeness is often equated with power, strength, confidence, and success—all positive male attributes. Male media attention also still tends to concentrate on the cerebral rather than the physical.

However, fashion is now taking an increasingly strong interest in male body image, with glossy adverts for men's fragrances displaying male torsos in all their toned glory. This development may be a factor in the growth of eating disorders among men, which account for about one in 10 cases of anorexia nervosa (0.2 percent of the male population). The true figure is probably much higher, since eating disorders are more difficult to diagnose in men and consequently go unreported. Also, as eating disorders are generally regarded as a woman's problem, men are less inclined to seek help.

In general, though, men are less likely than women to develop an eating disorder, partly because they are under less pressure to conform to a certain shape and partly because they have more lean body weight and less body fat. They are less likely to experience negative emotions about their weight or shape, and more likely to use exercise as a means of weight control than for dieting or purging.

Do Eating Disorders Start in Childhood?

Children today also are increasingly aware of body image and the pressure to conform to an ideal body shape. A study in 1993 by the Health Promotion Research Trust on 846 normal-weight 11- to 18-year-olds revealed that 70 percent of the girls thought they were fat, with many already dedicated dieters. Researchers at the Dublin Institute of Technology in 1994 found that out of one hundred 11-year-olds, 44 percent of the girls wanted to be lighter, despite the fact that most were of normal weight. In Australia, too, research has provided similarly alarming results, with 94 percent of school and university girls expressing a desire to be thinner, and 86 percent of those confessing to having dieted at least once.

It is therefore not surprising that the incidence of eating disorders among children is increasing rapidly; the Great Ormond Street Hospital in London reported a tenfold increase in child referrals from roughly 1984 to 1994. Growing numbers of young girls are attending slimming clubs and clinics, although a study at Kings College found that 32 percent of 12- to 16-year-old girls attending these diet clubs were not overweight.

When one considers children's role models, the current situation is not surprising. The toy industry's part in developing a child's attitude to body image should not be underestimated. The association between a perfect figure, beauty, and success is implanted in children's minds at an early age by dolls such as Barbie. Relative to the measurements of the average woman, Barbie's hips and waist are at least 10" smaller, the bust 8" smaller, and the inside leg 4" longer! Appealing cartoon creations such as the *Little Mermaid* also reinforce the attraction of this bizarre female shape.

Parents also play a vital part in shaping their children's attitudes to diet and body image. Psychologists find that mothers with a poor self-image and a preoccupation with dieting, weight, or fitness pass on a legacy of food and weight obsession to the next generation. With fundamental role models such as these, what sort of body image is the average 10-year-old going to have?

8

How Do Women Strive to Achieve the "Ideal" Body Shape?

Dieting among women is commonplace, with a study at Nottingham University finding that six out of ten women are dieting at any one time. If diets are monitored (e.g., by a reputable weight-loss club such as Weight Watchers), with weight loss and nutritional intake carefully observed, they can help one develop a healthier, fitter body. However, the restrictions and excessive self-control practiced by many dieters can give way to bouts of overindulgence, causing the dieter to feel guilty and thus resort to stricter control in the future. Inevitably, the dieter will lapse again, creating a vicious circle of yo-yo dieting. Food becomes an enemy rather than a necessary source of energy, and this distorted view may lead to disordered eating.

How Common Are Eating Disorders?

Recent figures from the Office of Health Economics (UK) show a disturbing increase in the incidence of anorexia nervosa and bulimia nervosa, with the number of sufferers doubling every decade. In the general population it is estimated that there are 125,000 bulimics and 70,000 anorexics. And it is thought that these figures represent only the tip of the iceberg since many cases are not reported. One study found that fewer than one-third of bulimics mentioned their eating disorder to their doctor.

What Is Anorexia Nervosa?

The term *anorexia nervosa* literally means "loss of appetite through nervous reasons." Typically, it begins in early adolescence but can develop at almost any age. Sufferers are in continual pursuit of a thin body and try to achieve this through starvation. They may begin with what appears to be a normal desire to lose weight, but as dieting continues, weight loss becomes an important achievement and they develop a more distorted body image, believing they are fat when they are in fact severely underweight. The fear of weight gain becomes an obsession. Many participate in exceptional levels of exercise to burn off extra calories and avoid fatness. They find it very difficult to acknowledge that they are ill and often withdraw socially, in part due to starvation and in part due a low feeling of self-worth.

What Causes Anorexia Nervosa?

There is no single cause in the development of anorexia nervosa. It is not simply a case of dieting gone awry, as it can be a means through which the individual attempts to deal with difficult emotional or psychological issues. Many researchers believe that media and cultural pressures on women to be thin are major contributing factors, but also that there are strong familial characteristics involved. Typically, the family of an anorexic places excessive emphasis on physical appearance, a need for approval, conformity, and high personal expectations, and measures self-worth and success by external standards.

What Are the Health Consequences of Anorexia Nervosa?

Anorexia nervosa can have serious physical and psychological consequences. Long-term food restriction inevitably results in an inadequate energy and nutrient intake. The initial signs include persistent fatigue due to depleted carbohydrate stores (glycogen). Low intakes of protein and carbohydrate lead to a breakdown of lean tissue (catabolism) and a decrease in tissue growth and repair (anabolism). An inadequate intake of vitamins and minerals means energy and nutrient metabolism may be compromised; for instance, a low intake of B vitamins can result in chronic fatigue. Reduced

Table 8.1: Characteristics and Warning Signs of Anorexia Nervosa

Characteristics	Warning signs
Severe weight loss	Extreme thinness and weight loss
Self-induced starvation	Excessive facial and body hair
Obsessive fear of weight gain	Claiming to be fat when thin
Feeling fat when thin	Eating very little
Low self-esteem	Great interest in food and calories
Social withdrawal	Anxiety and arguments about food
Obsessive exercise	Amenorrhea
Distorted body image	Feeling cold/bluish extremities
	Restless/sleeping very little
	Obsessive weighing

iron intake will result in depletion of existing iron stores and ultimately in iron deficiency anemia. Early symptoms include breathlessness upon mild exertion, impaired performance, and lightheadedness. Aerobic capacity (VO_2 max) is also reduced by as much as 28 percent.

The combination of low body weight, low body fat, poor nutrition, and excessive training leads to disturbances in the menstrual cycle and abnormal estrogen metabolism. Low estrogen levels associated with irregular or absent periods have been linked to reduced bone density and an increased risk of osteoporotic fractures.

Furthermore, anorexics often suffer gastrointestinal symptoms such as pain, bloating, constipation, and discomfort following eating. Hypotension (low blood pressure) and cardiac arrhythmia (heartbeat irregularities) also are common, while more severe complications such as heart muscle atrophy (wasting), slow heart beat, and abnormal liver and kidney function can also develop. Restricted fluid intake, which leads to chronic dehydration, is often exacerbated by further fluid losses due to self-induced vomiting or laxative/diuretic abuse. The most serious health consequence of anorexia nervosa is death. It has been estimated by the Eating Disorders Association that over 10 percent of sufferers die either from the disorder or by committing suicide.

Fortunately, many of the physical consequences of anorexia are reversible, and health can be restored through a good nutrition and weight-gain strategy. The psychological consequences are, however, more difficult to tackle. While some features, such as a preoccupation with food and a distorted body image, are more likely to *precede* the development of anorexia, others, such as difficulty in concentrating, social isolation, and self-centeredness, are more likely to result *from* the disorder. Anorexia itself exacerbates low self-esteem, fear of fatness, and the pursuit of thinness. There is some doubt as to whether these symptoms significantly decrease, even when the sufferer appears to have recovered physically. Researchers say that the personality characteristics associated with anorexia nervosa are very resistant to change: while the individual may change various aspects of her behavior, the basic personality tends to remain the same.

Health consequences of anorexia nervosa

- Reduced physical performance
- Decreased aerobic capacity
- Increased susceptibility to infections
- Slow recovery from injury
- Electrolyte imbalances
- Amenorrhea
- Cardiac arrhythmia
- Increased risk of bone loss and early osteoporosis
- Hypotension
- Hypothermia
- Gastrointestinal problems

Psychological characteristics of anorexia nervosa

- Preoccupation with food
- Fear of fatness
- Distorted body image
- Low self-esteem
- Depression and anxiety
- Perfectionism
- Obsessiveness
- High need for approval

Table 8.2: *Characteristics and Warning Signs of Bulimia Nervosa*

Characteristics	Warning signs
Bingeing on large amounts of food	Tooth decay/enamel erosion
Guilt and remorse after bingeing	Puffy face
Purging via vomiting/laxative abuse	Low weight or weight fluctuations
Starvation	Frequent weighing
Excessive exercise	Disappearing after meals to get rid of food
Distorted body image	Secretive eating
Obsession with food and weight	Menstrual disturbances

What Is Bulimia Nervosa?

Bulimia nervosa is characterized by compulsive binge eating, accompanied by self-induced vomiting, periods of starvation and excessive exercise, and purging with laxatives to avoid weight gain and alleviate guilt. Bingeing is usually secretive and preplanned, followed by enormous guilt and depression. Sufferers may consume up to 5,000 calories or more during one binge.

What Causes Bulimia Nervosa?

The disorder is likely to be triggered by a variety of difficult circumstances. It has been suggested that bulimics are predisposed to depression and that this can be exacerbated by a chaotic and conflicting family environment, a confused social role, and sometimes by sexual abuse. These factors lead to low self-esteem and an inability to face conflict or emotions. As with anorexia, media and cultural pressures to be thin also play a role, and the bulimic sees weight loss as a solution to her problems. Her ability to "cheat nature" by regulating her body shape by binge eating and purging allows her a measure of control over emotional confusion; the behaviors provide a temporary distraction for the sufferer from the real problem at hand. Emotions are thus suppressed and anxiety built up, to be released (at least partly) through bingeing and purging. A vicious cycle ensues, where bingeing and purging become a way to remove the guilt and shame associated with the acts as well as a way to avoid weight gain.

What Are the Health Consequences of Bulimia Nervosa?

Most of the health consequences of bulimia nervosa are due to the bingeing and purging rather than starvation, as in the case of anorexia nervosa. Menstrual irregularities are very common even when the individual's weight is normal. Amenorrhea is less likely than in anorexia nervosa.

Dental problems occur in bulimics who vomit, due to the action of the stomach acid, resulting in gum disease and erosion of tooth enamel. Gastrointestinal problems from vomiting or laxative abuse may include abdominal cramps, constipation, diarrhea, and, in extreme cases, ulceration and perforation of the esophagus or stomach lining.

Purging can result in dehydration and electrolyte imbalances, which in turn affect cardiovascular and renal functions. Other consequences include hypotension, lightheadedness, and poor circulation. Fortunately, many of the health consequences of bulimia nervosa (except tooth erosion) can eventually be reversed with a healthy nutritional program.

As with anorexia, many of the psychological characteristics of bulimia precede or are exacerbated by the development of the disorder. These include a low self-esteem, anxiety, depression, anger, a high need for approval, and mood swings. Most of these symptoms worsen with the severity and continuation of the disorder, and a vicious cycle develops as the bulimic symptoms make the sufferer feel even worse.

Health consequences of bulimia nervosa

- Menstrual irregularities
- Enamel erosion and gum disease
- Gastrointestinal problems
- Bowel problems
- Dehydration
- Electrolyte imbalances
- Cardiovascular complications
- Hypotension

Psychological characteristics of bulimia nervosa

- Food preoccupation

- Desire for thinness

- Low self-esteem

- Impulsiveness

- Depression, anxiety, anger

- Body dissatisfaction

- High need for approval

- Abnormal eating behavior

What Is Disordered Eating?

Although disordered eating is not a clinical eating disorder—it does not meet the American Psychiatric Association's (APA) official criteria for anorexia nervosa or bulimia nervosa—it does include some of the major symptoms of those diseases.

Sufferers have an intense fear of gaining weight or becoming fat, even though their weight is normal or (as is often the case) below normal. They are totally preoccupied with food and calories, having a fixation about their weight and a distorted body image. They attempt to lose weight by strict dieting, usually below 1,200 calories a day, and they exercise excessively. They have chaotic eating patterns and often have irregular or absent periods. Bingeing and purging are common, although the actual amount eaten during a "binge" is not much greater than a normal-sized meal; the sufferer simply perceives it to be excessive.

Health consequences of disordered eating

- Low energy levels

- Extreme fatigue

- Reduced performance

- Decreased aerobic capacity

- Increased susceptibility to infections

- Slow or poor recovery from injury

- Electrolyte imbalances

- Menstrual irregularities

- Amenorrhea

- Cardiovascular changes

- Increased risk of bone loss and early osteoporosis

- Depression

How Common Are Eating Disorders among Female Exercisers?

We have seen how the pressure to be thin affects women in general. To what extent is this situation reflected in the sports and fitness environment, where performance and physical achievement are considered paramount?

Disordered eating is so rife among female athletes and fitness participants that the term *anorexia athletica* is now applied in this respect. The extent of the problem is perhaps less surprising when one analyzes the shared psychological characteristics of individuals at risk of developing eating disorders and of elite athletes: competitiveness, perfectionism, compulsiveness, and a high degree of self-motivation are typical traits of both "personalities."

Sports and exercise give the athlete a sense of achievement and control over her body. Whereas in a confident, objective athlete this may be gained through the knowledge that she is in peak physical condition as a result of balancing her diet with the energy needs of her training program, for an athlete suffering from or predisposed to disordered eating, sports or fitness programs provide yet another means by which to lose weight or body fat. The prevalence of disordered eating in the sports and fitness environment is therefore not surprising.

Which Sports Are a Particular Cause for Concern?

The incidence of eating disorders is particularly high in sports that demand thinness, those where competition is fierce and where the sports environment (coaches/peers) and society exert pressure to conform to a certain body shape. While leanness can be a factor in improving performance in these areas, aesthetics are often given higher priority in restricting calorie intake. Gymnasts, ballet dancers, figure skaters, and long-distance runners are thus more prone to a distorted body image and eating disorders than women in sports where appearance is less important, for example, hockey, volleyball, basketball, and soccer.

Researchers at the University of North Texas conducted a survey of college gymnasts, with alarming results. Of the 215 gymnasts who completed detailed questionnaires, only 22 percent could be classified as having normal eating habits. Sixty-one percent had a subclinical eating disorder, and 16 percent had bulimia nervosa. The incidence of eating disorders among ballet dancers is also notoriously high. A study at Wolverhampton University found that two-thirds of ballet dancers were underweight, with a body mass index (BMI) below 20 (the normal range is 20–25).

This pattern is echoed, though to a lesser degree, in the male sports environment. Athletes considered most at risk include participants in weight-category sports such as wrestling, in sports such as long-distance running or horse racing, where weight affects performance, and in aesthetic sports such as bodybuilding.

Do Certain Sports Attract Women with an Eating Disorder?

The training programs of certain sports attract women who are prone to use excessive exercise as a means of losing or controlling weight. The positive relationship between leanness and performance in these areas legitimizes the athlete's pursuit of thinness, so that the sport provides an ideal camouflage for an athlete's illness, serving as a socially acceptable excuse to family and friends. In this respect, long-distance running is particularly appealing. Indeed, a recent survey of more than 4,000 recreational runners found that 24 percent of the women had attitudes suggestive of a serious eating disorder.

Do Certain Sports Cause Eating Disorders?

Researchers have looked at the possibility that the strenuous exercise regimens and restrictive diets required of certain sports can actually initiate anorexia nervosa. By suppressing the appetite and thereby decreasing food intake and body weight, the desire to exercise is increased. However, this theory assumes exercise as the focal point for the anorexia, whereas exercise in fact is often preceded by dietary restriction and weight loss. The theory also fails to explain bulimia nervosa.

What Effect Does an Eating Disorder Have on an Athlete's Performance?

Long-term food restriction can have serious physical consequences. Physical activity feels harder, fatigue occurs more readily, and performance is reduced. Recovery between training will be incomplete, and chronic fatigue (or "burnout"/overtraining) develops. The aerobic capacity (VO_2 max) will be dramatically reduced—by as much as 28 percent within 2 months of severe dieting—thereby canceling any performance "advantage" of a reduced body weight. An unbalanced diet can also result in low estrogen levels, increasing the risk of osteoporotic fractures. Indeed, as mentioned in Chapter 4, the British Olympic Medical Centre has recently reported a true osteoporotic fracture in a 30-year-old.

In summary, all of the physical consequences of eating disorders examined in this chapter combine to hinder performance and to drastically reduce the benefits of a training program.

How Does an Athlete with an Eating Disorder Continue Training?

It seems an extraordinary paradox that many sufferers continue to exercise and compete despite consuming far fewer calories than they expend. A number of studies, mainly of runners, have demonstrated large imbalances between energy intake and expenditure. Many competitive runners, for example, consume as few as 1,400 to 1,600 calories per day, barely enough to maintain their basal metabolic rate, let alone support their rigorous training. In one study of marathon runners who averaged 45 training miles per week, energy expenditure exceeded energy intake by more than 645 calories, yet their weights remained stable. Undoubtedly, a combination of psychological and physiological factors are involved.

On the physiological side, it has been suggested that the body adapts to the combination of excessive exercise and long-term restriction of calorie intake by becoming more energy efficient and reducing its metabolic activity. This would allow the athlete to train and to maintain energy balance and body weight on fewer calories than would be expected. Studies of nonathletes show that calorie restriction can lower basal metabolic rate by 10–30 percent. However, researchers have so far failed to agree on the combined effect of chronic dieting and exercise: some believe exercise prevents a drop in the metabolic rate, while others suggest that excessive exercise during dieting may slow it down.

To overcome physical and emotional fatigue, many anorexics and bulimics use stimulants such as caffeinated drinks (e.g., strong coffee and diet sodas) to give them energy. While this may initially boost performance, the effects will not last long, as depleted glycogen and nutrient stores will inevitably take their toll.

On the psychological side, the traits typical of the eating disorder "personality" (competitiveness, perfectionism, self-motivation, etc.) combine to lend the sufferer the impetus and strength to continue training, aided by the development of great stamina required to overcome the physical weaknesses incurred from restricted calorie intake.

The eating-disorders "personality"

- Obsessive
- Compulsive
- Perfectionist
- Self-motivated
- Competitive

"Personality" of elite athletes

- Dissatisfied with body shape

- Poor self-image

- Unhappy about appearance

- Distorted perception of body size

- More self-critical

- More emotionally reactive

Despite these physiological and psychological compromises, optimal performance cannot be sustained indefinitely. As glycogen and nutrient stores become chronically depleted, the athlete's health will suffer. Maximal oxygen consumption decreases, chronic fatigue sets in, and the athlete becomes more susceptible to injury and infection.

Some scientists believe, however, that many female athletes underreport their food intake and actually eat more than they admit. For example, a study at Indiana University of nine highly trained cross-country runners found that they were eating, on average, 2,100 calories per day, while their predicted energy expenditure was 3,000 calories. After analyzing the results of the Food Attitude Questionnaire, the researchers concluded that many had a poor body image and had inaccurately reported what they ate during the study.

How Should I Approach Someone Suspected of Having an Eating Disorder?

Approaching someone you suspect of having an eating disorder requires great care and sensitivity. Sufferers are likely to deny that they have a problem (anorexics often refuse to believe that they have a problem). They may feel embarrassed and their self-esteem threatened. Most fear that by admitting their problem they will be forced to gain weight or prevented from training or competing. Thus, it is vital to avoid direct confrontation about eating behavior or physical symptoms. The best person to approach the suspected sufferer is obviously someone with whom she has a close and trusting relationship.

8

The best strategy is usually to ask the sufferer how she feels and to let her know that you genuinely care. Be tactful and tread very gently. This may take several conversations over a long period of time. Do not suddenly present "evidence," such as observed weight loss, starving, bingeing, or purging, and avoid accusations or trying to "catch her" to prove your case. This will make her feel even more defensive and threatened, and will ultimately drive her further away from help.

What Should I Do if the Sufferer Admits She Has a Problem?

Getting the sufferer to admit to having an eating problem is a significant accomplishment in itself. Suggest that it would be best to have an initial consultation with an eating-disorders specialist. Help her make arrangements for a consultation as soon as possible, before she changes her mind.

Various forms of professional help are available. Some individuals may feel less threatened by talking to trained counselors from a self-help organization or a private eating-disorders clinic. A list of self-help organizations is given below. Others may feel comfortable with a doctor's referral, which usually involves treatment within a multidisciplinary team of psychologists and dietitians.

What Should I Do if the Sufferer Refuses to Admit a Problem?

If the sufferer initially denies she has a problem, drop the subject for 2 to 3 weeks before approaching it again. Don't push too hard at first. Repeated attempts may well be necessary, but avoid undue coercion. However, if she continues to deny the problem or refuse help and there is genuine concern for her health, a slightly more direct approach may be necessary. For example, ask her how much weight she has lost and then tactfully give information about a healthy weight for her sport. Ask about her menstrual cycle, and whether she feels fatigued, depressed, or irritable. Once she admits to any of these symptoms, carefully ask about her eating habits and let her know that you are concerned. Only as a very last resort, where there is great concern about her health, should you insist on a consultation with a physician or specialist.

What Type of Treatment Can the Sufferer Expect?

Different types of treatment are available, depending on the type and severity of the disorder and also on the sufferer herself. Bulimia nervosa is usually treated on an outpatient basis, whereas anorexia nervosa can involve a period of inpatient treatment.

The ultimate goal of treatment is to normalize weight and eating behavior, and to deal with the psychological issues that lie behind the eating disorder. The treatment for an anorexic patient involves restoring normal weight and health, as well as solving the problems that led to the initial development of the disorder. The treatment for a bulimic patient involves breaking the binge/purge cycle and developing a normal eating pattern.

Sufferers may receive individual psychotherapy with a qualified therapist who will determine the exact nature of the eating problem and develop an individual strategy for change. For anorexics, psychological changes often take years and require a great deal of honesty, trust, and sincerity. It may take many months before an anorexic patient will start to accept treatment, gain weight, and eat more.

Do you have an eating problem?

(This questionnaire is not intended as a diagnostic tool for eating problems, nor as a substitute for a full diagnosis by an eating-disorders specialist.)

- Do you exercise specifically to lose weight or fat?

- Do you worry about or dislike your body shape?

- Do you often "feel fat" one day and "thin" the next?

- Do your friends/family insist that you are slim while you feel fat?

- Do you feel guilty after eating a high-calorie or high-fat meal?

- Do you constantly scrutinize food labels to check the nutritional content?

- Do you avoid certain foods even though you want to eat them?

- Do you feel stressed or guilty if your normal diet or exercise routine are interrupted?

- Do you often decline invitations to meals and social occasions involving food in case you might have to eat something fattening?

Learning to break the habit

(This guide is not intended as treatment for an eating disorder. Treatment should always be sought from an eating-disorders specialist.)

- Learn to accept and like your body's shape—emphasize your good points.
- Realize that reducing your body fat will not solve deep-rooted problems or an emotional crisis.
- Don't set rigid eating rules for yourself and then feel guilty when you break them.
- Don't ban any foods or then feel guilty about eating anything.
- Establish a sensible, healthy eating pattern rather than a strict diet.
- Listen to your natural appetite cues—learn to eat when you are hungry.
- If you do overeat, don't try to "pay for it" later by starving yourself.
- Enjoy your exercise or sport for its own sake: have fun instead of enduring torture to lose body fat.

For bulimics, therapy usually lasts for about 20 sessions over 4 to 5 months. The first stage, which lasts about a month, involves establishing control over eating. The second stage, lasting about 2 months, involves changing the patient's attitude towards diet, eating behavior, and body shape, and increasing self-esteem. After this, a maintenance plan is made.

She may decide to join a self-help or support group, which will provide help from a therapist but also allow her to discuss her problem with and obtain support from fellow sufferers.

Sometimes family therapy is used, particularly for anorexic patients whose disorder developed before the age of 19. All of the family members are involved in the treatment. Here, the aim is to explore family relationships, dynamics, and issues that may have contributed to the eating disorder, and then to develop a family-based strategy to overcome the problem. Family therapy may be used in conjunction with inpatient behavioral therapy. Here, access to pleasurable activities or possessions is granted upon weight gain.

At some point in her treatment, the sufferer may be referred to a nutritionist or dietician for nutritional counseling. Although the sufferer often believes she is knowledgeable about food and eating behavior, she may actually have many misconceptions. The nutritionist or dietitian will be able to provide correct information and work out a nutritional program suited to the individual. She will provide reassurance about weight gain, encourage the recovering patient to eat in a variety of different settings, and can also counsel other members of the family about nutrition and eating habits.

═══Practical Points═══

■ Women generally have a more negative body image than men. They frequently overestimate their body size, are preoccupied with their weight, tend to aspire to unrealistic goals for weight loss, and are more likely than men to engage in destructive behavior to attain their ideal weight.

■ The fitness and sports environment puts women under great pressure to attain a low body weight and low body fat percentage. Those in "thinness demand" and weight-category sports tend to have a poorer body image.

■ Body dissatisfaction and preoccupation with size and shape often begins in adolescence and may be exacerbated by a number of other factors: mothers who themselves have a negative body image, peer pressure, perfectionist personality, media images of thinness, and pressure from coaches.

■ The desire to look lean or thin often exceeds the desire to win or train well. Many women take on excessive amounts of exercise in order to pursue their obsession with weight loss.

■ The athletic "personality" is often very similar to the eating-disorder "personality": obsessive, compulsive, perfectionist, and self-motivated.

- Women participating in fitness programs and sports are more likely to have a disordered pattern of eating than nonexercisers: it has been estimated that up to 60 percent have symptoms of a subclinical eating disorder.

- Anorexia nervosa is characterized by extreme thinness, self-induced starvation and weight loss, an intense fear of weight gain, feeling fat when thin, and amenorrhea.

- Bulimia nervosa is characterized by overconcern with body shape and weight, and frequent bingeing followed by guilt pangs, purging, starvation, or excessive exercise.

- Disordered eating is characterized by an intense fear of gaining weight or becoming fat (though the sufferer's weight may be within or below the normal range), distorted body image, excessive exercise for weight control, chaotic eating patterns, and a fixation with food and weight.

- Eating disorders and disordered eating patterns are more common in women involved in sports or activities requiring a very lean physique.

- It is unlikely that exercise itself causes eating disorders. Some women with a tendency to eating disorders are attracted to certain sports and exercise programs, and this environment may trigger the underlying disorder.

- Women should be encouraged to accept the fact that their natural, basic body shape cannot be changed by dieting or exercising.

- Less pressure to be thin should be placed on women by the media, the fashion industry, sports coaches, and judges.

- The physiological and psychological dangers of food restriction, dieting, and excessive exercise are not given enough attention; these should be highlighted more in the media, in gyms and health clubs, and through instructor/coach education.

- Women should not feel guilty about eating anything or "ban" any food from their diet. More emphasis should be placed on the enjoyment of eating so women can develop a healthy attitude towards food.

8

- Approaching someone with an eating disorder requires great care and sensitivity. Any direct confrontation about her symptoms or eating behavior should be avoided.

- If a sufferer admits to her problem, professional help should be sought from an eating-disorders specialist. Help is available from trained counselors and self-help organizations or via a doctor's referral.

Useful Organizations

National Institutes of Mental Health
(part of the National Institutes of Health)
(301) 443-4513/(301) 443-4536
www.nimh.nih.gov/publicat/eatingdisorder.cfm
(Alternatively, visit the home page at www.nih.gov; click on "Search"; type in "eating disorders.")

American Anorexia Bulimia Association, Inc. (AABA)
165 West 46th St., Ste. 1108
New York, NY 10036
(212) 575-6200
www.aabainc.org

Eating Disorder Awareness and Prevention, Inc. (EDAP)
603 Stewart St., Ste. 803
Seattle, WA 98101
(206) 382-3587 / Fax (206) 829-8501
www.edap.org

The National Eating Disorder Information Centre (NEDIC)
CW 1-211, 200 Elizabeth St.
Toronto, Ontario, Canada M5G 2C4
(416) 340-4156 / Fax (416) 340-4736
E-mail: nedic@uhn.on.ca
www.nedic.on.ca

═Further Reading═

T. A. Petrie, "Disordered Eating in Female Collegiate Gymnasts: Prevalence and Personality/Attitudinal Correlates" (*Journal of Sport and Exercise Psychology*, vol. 15, 1993, pp. 424–36).

K. A. Beals, M. M. Manore, "The Prevalence and Consequences of Subclinical Eating Disorders in Female Athletes" (*International Journal of Sports Nutrition*, vol. 4, 1994, pp. 175–95).

J. Sundgot-Bergon, "Eating Disorders in Female Athletes" (*Sports Medicine*, vol. 17, no. 3, 1994, pp. 176–88).

C. Davies, "Body Image, Dieting Behaviors and Personality Factors: A Study of High Performance Female Athletes" (*International Journal of Sports Psychology*, vol. 23, 1993, pp. 179–92).

T. A. Petrie, S. Stoever, "The Incidence of Bulimia Nervosa and Pathogenic Weight Control Behaviors in Female Collegiate Gymnasts" (*Quarterly Exercise Sport*, vol. 64, no. 2, 1993, pp. 238–41).

H. Saul, "Dying Swans?" (*New Scientist*, January 1994).

B. Dolan, I. Gitzinger, *Why Women? Gender Issues and Eating Disorders* (Athlone Press, 1994).

R. A. Thompson, R. Tattner Sherman, *Helping Athletes with Eating Disorders* (Human Kinetics Publishers, 1993).

R. West, *Eating Disorders: Anorexia Nervosa and Bulimia Nervosa* (Office of Health Economics, 1994).

T. Sanders, P. Bazalgette, *You Don't Have to Diet!* (Bantam Press, 1994).

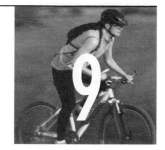

Competition Preparation: A Practical Guide

Peggy Wellington, B.Sc. (Hons), M.Phil.

Peggy Wellington, B.Sc., M.Phil., is a freelance sports nutritionist currently working as the nutrition consultant to the Amateur Swimming Association (UK) and national speed and figure skating squads, and is a member of the British Olympic Association's Nutrition Steering Group. She was a nutrition adviser at the 1992 Barcelona Olympic Games, 1993 World Athletic Championships, and 1994 Commonwealth Games, as well as numerous other international events. Codirector of P & A Sports Nutrition, she presents courses and seminars throughout Great Britain. A former track and field competitor, Peggy is in training to complete her first marathon.

The Chinese are said to drink caterpillar tea and turtle blood; the Kenyans prefer cow's blood. Countless athletes have devised their own special formulas to give them that ever-elusive "edge" over their opponents. There are endless stories of pre-event eating practices ranging from the extreme to the bizarre to the downright ridiculous! Tales of sprinters "carbo-loading" for extra energy, judo players starving themselves to shed those last few pounds, and swimmers tucking into curry and chips (because they swam fast last time they ate this meal) are not uncommon. Myths and misconceptions abound, and everyone has a horror story to tell when it comes to the competition diet. The end result is that many exercisers are confused about the ideal preparation for their particular activity.

This chapter evaluates the entire competition period by assessing the latest scientific recommendations and translating them into practical advice. And while this chapter concentrates on the physical aspects of preparation, the psychological implications of different eating patterns and food choices are also essential and should be considered at all times.

An athlete's preparation is not complete until she has considered the effects of her eating plan on the psychological and physical demands of her event. While the basic nutritional principles for male and female exercisers are essentially the same with regard to competition preparation, it is vital to consider event management so that women are fully aware of the importance of nutrition throughout the competition period.

What Should I Eat During the Week(s) Prior to an Event?

Your preparation will be dictated by the kind of event you are competing in, the importance of the event, and the frequency of competition. If you are performing a one-time sprint lasting only a few seconds, then dietary manipulation will have a limited effect. However, most competitions involve heats and finals or several rounds of competition on the same day. Fatigue in such events may be caused by glycogen depletion and/or dehydration. If you are participating in events involving prolonged, continuous exercise (for example, long-distance running, triathlon, or cycling) or multiple intervals of high-intensity activity (for example, swimming, basketball, soccer, squash, or tennis), then nutritional guidance may be crucial to your preparation.

Women competitors should aim to achieve the following nutrition goals:

- to ensure that liver and muscle glycogen stores are full
- to be well hydrated
- to avoid any new or unfamiliar practices that might negatively affect performance
- to "make weight" in sports such as judo and rowing without compromising performance
- to plan a nutrition strategy for the whole competition period—and be prepared to pack an "emergency food bag"!

How Can Liver and Muscle Glycogen Stores Be Optimally Filled?

An adequate taper (rest) in conjunction with a high-carbohydrate diet will ensure that glycogen stores are fully replenished. Generally, 24 to 48 hours of rest and a high-carbohydrate diet will allow adequate refueling. However, the presence of muscle damage will delay this process. Training that may cause muscle-fiber damage should either be scheduled earlier in the week to allow for recovery or be avoided altogether. Such training includes eccentric weight work, plyometric types of activity, hard running, and body contact sessions.

If competitions occur several times a week, as is the case in basketball and soccer, it may not be possible to rest for 48 hours prior to each event. Such a schedule would result in very little time to actually train. In this case, try to taper for the most important events. In addition, concentrate on lower intensity sessions or on skills/technique drills the day before the game rather than on a full-scale workout. The former is likely to cause a lesser degree of glycogen depletion.

How Much Carbohydrate Should Be Consumed During the Rest Period?

Your daily intake of carbohydrate during the 48-hour rest period should be as high as 9–10 grams per kilogram of body weight (divide weight in pounds by 2.2 to determine weight in kilograms). Since your training diet should already be high in carbohydrate, the only change for many athletes will be the rest from training. If your normal diet contains much less carbohydrate than this, gradually increase the quantity that you are eating during the days leading up to the event.

Table 9.1: Recommended Daily Carbohydrate Intake in Preparation for Competition

Body weight	Range of daily carbohydrate intake (9–10 g/kg)
40 kg (88 lbs.)	360–400 g
50 kg (110 lbs.)	450–500 g
60 kg (132 lbs.)	540–600 g
70 kg (154 lbs.)	630–700 g
80 kg (176 lbs.)	720–800 g

For some women, 9–10 g/kg/day may seem like a huge quantity of carbohydrate. However, such large intakes are necessary to ensure the efficient and complete replenishment of glycogen.

Use Table 9.1 to check how much carbohydrate to eat during the rest days before a competition, and refer to Chapter 1 for information on which foods to eat. Table 9.1 should be used only as a guide, since individual circumstances may require you to consume more or less carbohydrate than recommended here. Although it may seem less than scientific, experimenting with your training regimen, simulated competitions, and minor events is often the most effective way to find out what works best for you.

Put another way, if your event lasts for less than 90 minutes, your training diet—which should provide 60 percent of energy from carbohydrate, or 9–10 g/kg/day—coupled with adequate rest will ensure that you have enough fuel on board to last you for the entire event. If, however, your event lasts for longer than 90 minutes, you may want to consider carbohydrate loading (see below) to boost your carbohydrate intake to up to 70 percent of your calorie intake—or more than 10 g/kg/day.

Menu Guides

The three menus found in Table 9.2 are designed to supply a carbohydrate intake of approximately 400 g, 600 g, and 800 g. They are ideal for use during the 2 to 3 days prior to a major competition. *Note: Although they meet the requirements for carbohydrate, they are extremely low in fat and therefore may not necessarily be suitable for everyday use.*

In some cases, you may discover that you will need to consume more carbohydrate and that your training diet does not meet the recommendations above. If additional carbohydrate is required over and above your everyday intake, follow the guidelines given in Table 9.3.

Beware of increasing the amount of fat that you are eating. It is easy to get carried away so that in an attempt to boost the carbohydrate content of your diet the fat intake creeps up as well! In fact, fat consumption during a taper period should be further reduced to ensure that your calorie intake remains the same. Otherwise you may experience a gain in weight.

This becomes essential during a taper that lasts longer than a few days. A corresponding decrease in energy intake should be planned to match the reduced workload. Calories should be reduced by eating less fat.

Table 9.2: *Menus That Provide Varying Levels of Carbohydrate Intake*

400 g carbohydrate from:	600 g carbohydrate from:	800 g carbohydrate from:
Breakfast Cornflakes (large bowl) with sugar and skim milk Chopped banana with raisins ½ pint fruit juice	*Breakfast* 2 bananas on 4 slices of toast 1 pint fruit juice	*Breakfast* Sweetened cereal (large bowl) with skim milk Scone or low-fat muffin (with small pat of butter) Handful of grapes 1 pint fruit juice
Snack 1 apple	*Snack* 1 Pop Tart	*Snack* 1 pint chocolate or strawberry milk (low-fat) 2 pancakes with syrup
Lunch Turkey-breast sandwich with lettuce and tomato (2 slices of bread, no butter or mayonnaise) Low-fat yogurt 1 orange 1 pint diluted fruit juice	*Lunch* Medium deep-pan pizza (ham and pineapple or other low-fat option) with salad Low-fat yogurt 1 pear ½ pint diluted fruit juice	*Lunch* 2 bagels with ½ cup hummus spread Bowl of jello with fruit ½ pint diluted fruit juice
Snack Scone and jam (no butter)	*Snack* 1 bagel with low-fat cream cheese or hummus spread	*Snack* Bowl of sweetened cereal with skim milk 1 banana
Dinner Large baked potato (no butter) Low-fat cottage cheese with tuna filling Large salad (fat-free dressing) Fresh or canned fruit	*Dinner* Large plate rice (100 g dry weight) Small portion chili con carne (150 g) Corn and peas Yogurt, banana, and dry cereal ½ pint fruit juice	*Dinner* Large portion pasta (100 g dry weight) Meat sauce (150 g) Broccoli and carrots Fruit crisp (low-fat) ½ pint diluted fruit juice
	Nighttime snack Low-fat yogurt	*Nighttime snack* 2 slices of toast with small pat of butter Honey
ALSO 1 liter isotonic-type sports drink throughout the day 2,000 calories (8,400 kilojoules) 74% of calories = carbohydrate 13% = fat 13% = protein	*ALSO* 1 liter diluted fruit juice throughout the day 3,400 calories (14,280 kilojoules) 66% of calories = carbohydrate 23% = fat 11% = protein	*ALSO* 1 liter diluted fruit juice throughout the day 4,000 calories (166,800 kilojoules) 75% of calories = carbohydrate 14% of calories = fat 11% = protein

Table 9.3: A Practical Guide to Boosting the Carbohydrate Content of Your Diet
in Preparation for Competition

- Reduce the fat and protein component of the meal and add extra carbohydrate. For example, have an extra potato and less meat, an extra spoonful of rice or pasta and a spoonful less of oily/creamy sauce.
- Choose a thick-crust pizza rather than a thin one, but cut down on the fatty toppings, i.e., more sauce, vegetables, tuna, and pineapple, and less cheese.
- Drink extra juices or sports drinks with your meals. This adds additional carbohydrate with no extra fat.
- Add dried fruit, chopped banana, or sugar to breakfast cereal.
- Add sugar to hot drinks.
- Choose high-carbohydrate, low-fat snacks, such as dried fruit, sweetened popcorn (not buttered), jello, hard candies, dried breakfast cereal, fat-free crackers, bananas.

At no time should you reduce the carbohydrate content of your diet. Remember, excess dietary fat is very efficiently stored as fat.

Finally, there is no need to stuff yourself to the point of discomfort. A successful regimen will involve eating small to moderate high-carbohydrate, low-fat meals and snacks to meet the recommendations given in Table 9.1.

Remember:

- to maintain hydration at all times by drinking plenty of fluids;
- to stick to a familiar nutrition program and avoid any new, untried practices or foods which may negatively affect your performance; and
- to think ahead and predict any problems which might occur. Always be prepared to take food with you, particularly if you are staying away from home or traveling abroad.

What About Weight-Class Sports?

Weight-control sports may pose additional problems. Traditional methods of making weight include restriction of food and fluids and the use of sweat suits, saunas, laxatives, and diuretics. Clearly such methods will compromise performance due to a combination of reduced glycogen levels and dehydration.

Safe, effective weight loss that does not negatively affect perform-ance can only be achieved by a gradual reduction in fat consumption. This in turn will lead to a reduction in body-fat content. This strategy will involve planning to "make weight" weeks before the start of the competition and not at the last minute, as is often the case.

Carbohydrate and fluid intake must be maintained at all times in order to support the training load. A reduction in carbohydrate intake will lead to an inability to train and compete properly as a result of reduced glycogen stores. Similarly, dehydration can reduce exercise capacity and adversely affect performance.

A major problem with increasing the carbohydrate content of the diet in the week prior to the event is that the extra carbohydrate, stored with water as glycogen, causes you to weigh more. While this extra glycogen is an advantage for most women, it can be a disadvantage in weight-dominated sports, where the category is often reached by the narrowest of margins.

This highlights the importance of forward planning so that weight is made in advance and the athlete is able to maintain a high-carbohydrate diet accompanied by plenty of fluids. The advantage of such preparation is obvious, and any athletes who follow this strategy will be at a huge advan-tage over their competitors.

What Is Carbohydrate Loading?

Carbohydrate loading is the term used to describe the elevation above nor-mal levels of muscle glycogen levels. It is sometimes referred to as super-compensation.

The traditional or "classical" regimen involves completing an ex-hausting training session followed by a low-carbohydrate, high protein, and high-fat diet. This depletion phase is maintained for 3 to 4 days in order to increase the levels of the enzyme responsible for storing glycogen in the muscle. If the muscle is then "crammed" with plenty of carbohydrate—if, that is, the individual switches to an extremely high-carbohydrate diet—then additional glycogen is stored.

In practice, such a regimen is unpleasant to follow. Problems fre-quently occur during the depletion phase, when athletes may experience fatigue and gastrointestinal upsets from the high-protein, high-fat diet. They may also suffer mood swings and irritability. Despite this, many athletes ranging from sprinters to ultra-distance runners confess to having tried carbohydrate loading.

Is It Possible to Carbohydrate Load Without a Depletion Phase?

The simple answer is yes. In light of the problems associated with such a regimen, American researchers have developed a modified glycogen-loading program that is as effective as the classical method and can increase muscle glycogen stores as much as 20 to 40 percent above normal.

The modified program is similar to the normal preparation for competition except that the rest period is extended and slightly more carbohydrate is consumed.

On days seven to four prior to the event, a normal mixed diet should be eaten. This will typically contain less carbohydrate than you are used to eating (approximately 50 percent of caloric intake). Training should be moderately hard (1 to 2 hours per day). Three days before the event, training should be reduced to no more than 60 minutes of low-intensity work accompanied by a carbohydrate intake of *at least* 9 to 10 g/kg/day (or up to 70 percent of energy).

Since this scheme will almost certainly require you to consume more carbohydrate than normal, follow the guidelines given in Table 9.3 for some ideas. A word of caution, however: don't get carried away and end up fat-loading as well! Focus your food choices on high- carbohydrate, low-fat meals and snacks. Fluid intake should remain high at all times.

Carbohydrate loading is mainly relevant in events involving over 90 minutes of continuous, high-intensity activity that stresses the same muscle groups. Such exercise will challenge the athlete's normal fuel stores. There is, however, a small amount of evidence that indicates that carbohydrate loading may also improve performance during maximal exercise which only lasts several minutes.

If you have experienced a drop in pace or a reduction in performance in conjunction with feelings of muscle-glycogen depletion towards the end of an event, then you may benefit from this procedure. Always experiment in a minor competition or under simulated event conditions to ensure that it works for you. Never try it for the first time in preparation for an important competition.

What Should Be Eaten for the Precompetition Meal?

Traditionally it was believed that a high-protein meal would set you up for the day's events. It is still common to hear reports of football players tucking into steak, eggs, and fries prior to a game. This type of meal offers little in the way of carbohydrate and is less than ideal for the nutrition-conscious competitor.

The aims of the pre-event meal are to top up glycogen stores (muscle glycogen stores should already be full if you have organized your preparation well, but liver glycogen stores may need replenishing), to maintain hydration, to stave off hunger, and to give the competitor a psychological boost.

Foods ingested during this period should be high in carbohydrate and low in fat since high-fat foods are digested more slowly. They should also be low in fiber and bulk. This is particularly important for athletes who are prone to pre-event nerves, diarrhea, or "the trots." Always choose foods that are well tolerated and have a high to moderate glycemic index (see Chapter 1) to ensure rapid digestion and absorption.

Research suggests that performance can be improved when a carbohydrate-rich meal is consumed 3 to 4 hours before prolonged exercise. In one particular study, cyclists improved their power output by 22 percent when they consumed 200 g of carbohydrate from bread, cereals, and fruit 4 hours prior to exercising, as well as a chocolate bar (43 g of sucrose) 5 minutes before exercise. This is because a relatively large pre-exercise meal appears to increase performance by maintaining a high use of carbohydrate later on in endurance exercise.

Lesser amounts of carbohydrate (i.e., 50–150 g) have not produced the same responses.

Practically, however, 200 g of carbohydrate can be bulky to consume! Some women may not be able to tolerate this quantity of carbohydrate even if some of it is in fluid form.

Table 9.4: Pre-event Meals and Snacks

Breakfast cereal and low-fat/skim milk
Toast (small pat of butter) with honey/jam
Banana or jam sandwiches
Low-fat muffins with jam/honey
Pancakes and syrup
Hummus on bagels
Pasta with tomato-based sauce
Baked potato with low-fat topping
Canned or fresh fruit
Low-fat rice pudding
Scones with jam
Whole-grain crackers and low-fat/skim milk

The essential thing is that the meal should not cause any discomfort or feelings of bloatedness. As a result, the timing of the meal and quantity of food eaten will vary from individual to individual despite the fact that studies recommend ingesting 200–300 g of carbohydrate during the 4 hours prior to exercise.

The key is to find out what works for you and then to stick to it. As a general rule, if a large meal is consumed, then leave 3 or 4 hours for it to digest. If you consume a pre-event snack, then leave 1 to 2 hours. If you are involved in a sport that requires a weigh-in, then you will probably leave your pre-event meal until afterwards.

Some ideas for pre-event meals and snacks are listed in Table 9.4. These should always be accompanied by some fluid.

If solid foods cannot be tolerated during this time, then use liquid meals such as carbohydrate supplements (e.g., Twin Labs Carbo Fuel, Power Bar Gel, Optimum's Carbo Pump and Carb Xcelerator) or sports drinks (e.g., Powerade, Gatorade, Twin Labs Ripped Fuel, Optimum's Pro Complex Drink and Amino Xcelerator), high-carbohydrate baby foods, or crackers with low-fat milk or jelly.

It is vital to continue to drink fluids right up to the start of your first event. Carry a water bottle with you at all times and choose sports drinks, diluted juices, or water.

Remember: choose white bread and lower-fiber cereals, and avoid high-fiber foods such as beans if you suffer from any intestinal or bowel problems, unless you are sure that you can tolerate them

If you find that you become hungry prior to the event's start, then have a small, carbohydrate-rich snack. Ignoring hunger pangs will cause you to focus on your stomach rather than on the competition—so have something to eat!

Should Sugary Products Be Consumed Within 1 Hour of an Event?

Many athletes believe that sugar consumption should be avoided prior to exercising. The belief arises from suggestions that such a practice may upset blood sugar levels and suppress the metabolism of fatty acids, ultimately causing glycogen to be used more quickly than normal.

These recommendations appear to arise from one or two studies—conducted as long ago as 1977—which reported a negative effect after ingesting sugar just prior to performance. Subsequent studies have failed to reproduce these results. Some have demonstrated no effect of sugar intake on performance, but interestingly, more recent work has suggested that sugar ingestion may have an ergogenic effect by actually enhancing performance. The suggested mechanisms for this improvement in performance in endurance events is that the sugar provides extra carbohydrate either to support high rates of carbohydrate oxidation or to maintain blood sugar levels later on in exercise. In any case, substantial evidence exists to show that even if blood sugar levels are disturbed, metabolism reverts back to its normal pattern once exercise has started, with no adverse effect on performance.

Recent reports lead us to conclude, therefore, that there is little support for the idea that sugar ingestion prior to performance actually impairs performance. Indeed, there is growing evidence to suggest that this may be a useful practice in events where glycogen depletion is a problem.

A recent study by a group of Spanish researchers indicates that feeding a glucose drink (75 g) to runners 30 minutes prior to a run of high intensity and intermediate duration can significantly improve the time to exhaustion compared with drinking plain water or fructose. This suggests that the advantages of sugar feeding prior to performance may not be limited to prolonged events.

Anyone who believes that they may benefit from a small, sugar-rich snack (approximately 50 g) prior to exercise should experiment in training or minor competitions first. Anecdotal evidence suggests that exercisers tolerate the carbohydrate better in the form of fluid confectionery (for example, chocolate, jelly babies, jelly beans, or energy bars).

What about Fluid Intake?

Dehydration will impair exercise capacity and can cause serious risks to health. Dehydration may impair performance when as little as 2 percent of body weight is lost through sweating (i.e., 1.2 kg for a 60 kg [132 lbs.] female). It is essential that hydration is maintained at all times throughout a competition, even if you are involved in an activity which requires you to "make weight."

Weight and urine checks provide practical ways to monitor your fluid status. A weight reduction of 1 kg is the equivalent of 1 liter of sweat lost. A simple "before the event" and "after the event" weight check can help you to determine your fluid requirements. In addition, frequent visits to the toilet and the production of copious quantities of pale-colored urine indicates adequate hydration. In contrast, a lesser quantity of dark-colored, smelly urine indicates dehydration.

During short, high-intensity events such as sprinting, middle-distance track events, competitive swimming events, judo bouts, and other exercise periods lasting up to 30 minutes, it is not usually necessary, nor is it often possible, to consume fluid during the event. This is presuming that the competitor is well hydrated prior to the event's start and continues to compensate for fluid losses between bouts of exercise. However, it is difficult to identify a cut-off point beyond which fluid consumption becomes essential, since many factors will influence the individual's requirements.

If exercise is of a longer duration, fluid replacement during exercise is usually necessary since sweat losses can be high and there is a real risk of dehydration if fluid is not consumed.

Opportunities to take fluid on board should be organized during longer events. Drinks breaks should be scheduled, and competitors should make use of any available opportunity to consume some fluid. This is particularly important during events where the rules dictate the opportunity to drink—for example, in many team games.

The amount of fluid that is drunk will depend on a number of factors. During prolonged activity where large sweat losses are predicted, it is recommended that fluid is ingested before, during, and after exercise at regular intervals. It is recommended to start the event with the maximum quantity of fluid tolerable in your stomach. This should be topped up during the activity.

A fluid intake of 150–250 ml (6 to 8 fluid ounces) per 15 minutes is often recommended, although problems are clearly associated with making such hard and fast rules. The key is to practice drinking and to offset weight losses of more than 1 percent of your total body weight.

What Drinks Are Recommended?

A dilute carbohydrate-electrolyte drink will deliver water faster to the tissues than plain water. This is because small amounts of glucose and sodium stimulate the uptake of water in the intestine. Hence the reason why some sports drinks (such as Isostar and Gatorade) are formulated to contain both these ingredients.

Consumption of a well-formulated sports drink during prolonged, high-intensity exercise (1 to 3 continuous hours) when sweat losses are high is essential to ensure that fluid needs are met.

In shorter events, where sweat losses are not significant, a number of drinks are suitable, such as water or diluted fruit juice. It is unlikely that fluid or fuel deficits will be serious in shorter events. However, it is prudent to err on the side of caution and to take fluid on board just in case.

During the Event—Food or Fluid?

Sports drinks have the added advantage of containing a substantial quantity of carbohydrate (between 50 and 80 g/liter). As a result they can meet the dual requirements for energy and fluid during exercise.

Carbohydrate feedings during an event appear to be of little benefit in activities that are not limited by carbohydrate availability. Such events include sprint swimming and running, baseball, and figure skating.

However, carbohydrate feeding during prolonged exercise has been shown to delay fatigue by preventing hypoglycemia and maintaining high rates of glucose use. The effects of such feedings are clear in cyclists but less obvious in running events. Since the amount of carbohydrate available later in exercise will influence performance, it seems reasonable to suggest that it may be of benefit to consume carbohydrate in events of a continuous nature that last longer than 60 minutes.

Research undertaken in the 1990s has also indicated that a carbohydrate drink consumed during prolonged exercise may help to maintain white-cell functioning; this might in turn reduce the risk of becoming ill once the exercise is over. Further research is required to substantiate this.

If glycogen stores are reduced prior to the start of the exercise (a situation that is common among participants), then carbohydrate supplementation will have a more immediate effect.

During extreme activities such as road races, triathlon, ultra-distance running, sailing, and distance rowing, athletes may also desire food. This can contribute to an increased carbohydrate intake. Foods with a high glycemic index should be selected and be accompanied by fluid. Common choices include:

- energy bars, candy bars, and cereal/granola bars
- raisins and bananas
- sugar confectionery (i.e., pastry, candy)
- jello cubes
- sandwiches
- Pop Tarts
- canned fruit

Carbohydrate feedings are also of benefit in high-intensity, intermittent activities such as soccer, hockey, basketball, and tennis. Such exercises are glycogen depleting, so the benefits may be due to the glycogen-sparing effects of the feedings.

How Much Carbohydrate Should Be Consumed During Exercise?

Research suggests that sufficient carbohydrate should be consumed to supply approximately 1 g/minute. Many of the studies in this area have used protocols that involved feeding subjects between 30–60 g carbohydrate per hour to produce an ergogenic effect. Researchers from the University of Maastrict in The Netherlands showed that the ingestion of 50 g of carbohydrate at the start of exercise followed by 12–13 g each 15 minutes led to near maximal rates of oxidation of these carbohydrate supplements during a 2-hour cycle exercise.

The 30–60 g/hour range should be used only as a guideline; individual intakes should be adapted more specifically to the athlete's circumstances. Trial and error and a bit of logic will help to determine exactly how much carbohydrate is needed.

One liter of an isotonic-type sports drink will supply approximately 70 g of carbohydrate. Therefore, the regular consumption of a sports drink, starting early in exercise, provides a convenient method of meeting both fluid and carbohydrate needs.

What About All-day Events?

Competitions often last all day, and may continue for several days. In such tournament situations women may be competing several times each day with variable amounts of rest between bouts of exercise. The question always arises as to what to eat and drink between sessions. Food choices will be influenced by several factors, including the length of time between events, food availability, and individual preferences. However, women should use these breaks to top up glycogen stores and replenish fluid levels.

As a general rule, when there is less than one hour between events it is wise to stick to sports drinks and fruit drinks. Food intake may be a problem due to the limited time for digestion and absorption and the possibility of gastric discomfort. Having said this, some competitors may choose to eat a light carbohydrate snack at this time.

Table 9.5: *Guidelines for Eating at All-day Events*

Less than one hour	Two to four hours
Sports drinks (e.g., Twin Labs Ripped Fuel, Gatorade, Powerade)	Sandwiches/rolls/pita bread
Carbohydrate supplements (e.g., Twin Labs Carbo Fuel, Power Bar Gel, Optimum's Carbo Pump and Carb Xcelerator)	Bagels/muffins/ scones/pancakes
	Toast/toasted sandwiches
	Cereal/crackers
Diluted fruit juice	Pop Tarts
	Popcorn
	Canned or dried fruit
Possibly:	Low-fat rice pudding
Bananas and raisins	Pasta with tomato sauce
Energy bars	Baked potato with low-fat topping
Candy (e.g., jelly beans)	Rice with low-fat sauce
Jello cubes	
Plain crackers	*Remember:*
Rice cakes	*Keep drinking at all times!*
	Keep the fat content of the meal low!
	Do not stuff!
	Eat small amounts and often.

If there are 2 to 4 hours between events, a light, carbohydrate-rich meal will help to begin to restore glycogen to its preexercise levels.

Use Table 9.5 to identify ideas for snacks and meals.

Is There a Special Postcompetition Strategy?

Once the competition has completely finished, then it is time to celebrate and to give yourself a well-deserved rest. If, however, you are competing the following day or within the next few days, your postevent food intake is crucial.

Muscle glycogen resynthesis is faster than normal immediately after exercise. Women should aim to take some carbohydrate on board (approximately 1 g/kg) as soon after exercise as is practical. This will probably be in the form of fluid or a carbohydrate-rich snack.

This should be followed by a carbohydrate-rich meal consumed approximately 2 hours later. Some research has shown that muscle glycogen resynthesis may be near optimal when at least 50 g of carbohydrate is consumed at 2-hour intervals.

Studies done in the 1990s at Ohio State University propose a strategy that may increase the rate of glycogen storage by up to 20 percent over and above the 50 g/2 hours regimen outlined above. The study involved exhaustive exercise that severely reduced the subject's muscle glycogen levels. Following each workout, subjects consumed carbohydrate every 15 minutes for 4 hours! This pattern of eating is sometimes called grazing. The amount of carbohydrate consumed was enormous—almost 3 grams per pound of body weight or 6 g per kg of body weight (more than many people consume in a day, and over half the daily recommendation for individuals in heavy training)! This was then subdivided into 16 equal doses over the 4-hour period, so that the athletes were ingesting about 30 g of carbohydrate every 15 minutes. Imagine eating two bananas or drinking 500 ml (one pint) of sports drink every 15 minutes for 4 hours after exercise!

Muscle biopsies revealed that 20 percent more glycogen was stored than when 50 g of carbohydrate was consumed every 2 hours.

It is possible that this 15-minute strategy is so effective because it ensures high blood glucose and insulin levels over a 4-hour period, therefore enhancing glycogen storage.

Before you rush out to try this plan, it must be stressed that the subjects had participated in *exhaustive* exercise prior to the "loading" program. It is likely that such a scheme will only be relevant for women who are involved in activities that are severely glycogen depleting.

It may be a useful strategy to employ during periods of intensive training or if you are competing more than once a day. As with all these programs, it may not be suitable for everyone and must be tried and tested in training first. From a practical viewpoint it may be impossible for a person to consume that amount (over half your daily requirement) of carbohydrate in the space of 4 hours. Such schemes should be carefully planned with the help of a qualified sports nutritionist.

A modified version of this plan—and one that would be easier to achieve from a practical point of view—involves consuming the recommended post-event carbohydrate-rich snack, then continuing to consume fluid (containing some carbohydrate) until a meal is consumed. In this way a continuous stream of carbohydrate is supplied to the muscles.

═══Practical Points ═══

- Taper your training and maintain a high-carbohydrate diet (9–10 g/kg body weight) in the days prior to a competition to ensure maximal storage of glycogen.

- Women involved in events where carbohydrate availability is a limiting factor may benefit from carbohydrate loading.

- Drink plenty of fluids to offset dehydration.

- Avoid practices that cause dehydration or glycogen depletion to make a weight category.

- Ensure that pre-event meals and snacks are carbohydrate-rich, and low in fat, fiber, and bulk.

- Drink before, during (if relevant), and after the event.

- Top up glycogen stores with suitable high-carbohydrate foods and drinks during the event (where necessary) and between events.

- Ensure that you follow an adequate refueling and rehydration plan if competing on subsequent days.

- Never try anything new during the period before an event. Stick to a tried and tested regimen.

- Try out new ideas and plans in training or at less important events.

- Plan ahead and always pack suitable snacks and drinks in your bag.

- If you have any doubts about your preparation, then consult a qualified sports nutritionist.

Further Reading

F. Brouns, *Nutritional Needs of Athletes* (John Wiley & Sons, 1993).

D. L. Costill, M. Hargreaves, "Carbohydrate Nutrition and Fatigue" (*Sports Medicine*, vol. 13, 1992, pp. 86–92).

J. Fallowfield, C. Williams, "Carbohydrate Intake and Recovery from Prolonged Exercise" (*International Journal of Sports Nutrition*, vol. 3, 1993, pp. 150–64).

"Food Nutrition and Sports Performance: Proceedings of an International Scientific Consensus" (*Journal of Sports Sciences*, vol. 9, special issue, Summer 1991).

"Foods, Nutrition and Soccer Performance: Proceedings of an International Scientific Consensus" (*Journal of Sports Sciences*, vol. 12, special issue, Summer 1994).

P. D. Neufer, et al., "Improvements in Exercise Performance: Effects of Carbohydrate Feedings and Diet" (*Journal of Applied Physiology*, vol. 63, 1987, pp. 983–88).

J. G. Seifert, et al., "Glycemic and Insulinemic Response to Preexercise Carbohydrate Feedings" (*International Journal of Sport Nutrition*, vol. 4, no. 1, March 1994).

J. L. Ventura, et al., "Effect of Prior Ingestion of Glucose or Fructose on the Performance of Exercise of Intermediate Duration" (*European Journal of Applied Physiology*, vol. 68, 1994, pp. 345–49).

A. J. M. Wagenmakers, et al., "Oxidation Rates of Orally Ingested Carbohydrates During Prolonged Exercise" (*Journal of Applied Physiology*, vol. 75, no. 6, December 1994, pp. 2774–80).

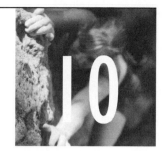

Making Weight

Jane Griffin

Jane Griffin qualified from London University with a degree in Nutrition and a Post-graduate Diploma in Dietetics. After working for several years in industry for a variety of food and pharmaceutical companies, she set up her own nutritional and dietetic consultancy 12 years ago. She has specialized in spreading the "health eating" message via media work with women's magazines, radio, and television. Over the last 8 years she has also become more and more involved in the area of sports nutrition. She is the Consultant Nutritionist to the British Olympic Association and traveled with the Great Britain team to the Barcelona Olympic Games in 1992. Jane has written for Running *magazine and* Squash Player *for several years, as well as for* Athletics Weekly, Martial Arts Today, *and* Performance Cyclist. *She now writes for* Karate World *and the* Bike Mag.

Most female athletes find that they perform best at a particular body weight or at least within a narrow range of body weights. For some athletes, however, their sport dictates that they must compete at a particular weight—one that is seldom their natural one. As a result, they have to lose weight.

This is usually done by making weight, so called because an athlete must weigh a certain amount in order to "make" a weight class prior to competition. Such sports include martial arts, weightlifting, wrestling, and lightweight rowing. Other athletes, such as body builders, dancers, and figure skaters, may need to make weight to improve appearance, while gymnasts and jockeys may lose weight close to competing by dehydration in the hope of increasing stamina and power relative to body weight.

Weight classes are determined by the particular sport's governing body. In the case of lightweight rowing, women row at a maximum body weight of 59 kg with an average crew weight of 57 kg. In other sports, weight classes are intended to eliminate injuries that could arise if competitors were ill-matched physically, or to allow athletes of all sizes to compete on an equal basis. Unfortunately, it does not necessarily work like that. Many athletes lose weight to qualify for a lower weight class in the belief that they will have the advantage of size, strength, power, and leverage over their opponent. To gain competitive advantage, they seek to compete at a weight where the power-to-weight ratio is optimal, where muscle mass is maximized and body fat minimized.

How Is Weight Made?

Athletes use various methods to make weight. Some keep their body weight continually low by following a strict diet year round. Others lose weight during the season and gain it back during off-season, while still others gain and lose weight repeatedly throughout the season and from season to season. Athletes in general, but the latter group in particular, also use a variety of methods to lose weight. They include:

- *Food restriction*—severe reduction in total energy (calorie) intake

- *Starvation*—complete avoidance of food for one or more days before weigh-in

- *Fluid restriction*—rationing or complete avoidance of fluid intake one or more days before weigh-in

- *Heat exposure*—use of saunas, steam rooms, and hot showers to encourage weight loss by dehydration through sweating

- *Strenuous exercise*—long, hard training sessions to encourage weight loss by dehydration through sweating. Sweat rate is often increased by wearing extra clothing—track suits, wool hats and scarves, or sweat suits—during the session

- *Diuretics*—to stimulate the kidneys to produce more urine, increase fluid losses, and therefore increase weight loss

- *Vomiting and laxatives*—to ensure that the stomach is empty and that all waste products are removed, thus making the body as "light" as possible

What Are the Problems Involved with Making Weight?

The basic principles of making weight are either to cut back food intake so severely that the body has to call on its own stores to supply the energy deficit, or to reduce the body's total water content by dehydration or restriction of fluid intake. Both practices can affect health and performance, depending on the severity and frequency of their use.

What Are the Problems of a Restricted Food Intake?

Although the aim is to reduce energy or calorie intake, restricting food intake overall also reduces—sometimes dangerously so—the intake of essential nutrients such as vitamins, minerals, carbohydrates, and proteins.

- *Carbohydrate*—strict dieting or starvation causes a fall in muscle and liver glycogen levels, resulting in fatigue and poor performance, particularly in endurance events such as rowing. In other sports the effect may be cumulative during a competition and become apparent as an athlete advances through the rounds. Complete replenishment of severely depleted muscle glycogen stores can take up to 48 hours.

- *Protein*—in a similar way, protein intake may be inadequate for athletic performance. Recent research suggests that strength or speed athletes should consume about 1.2–1.7 g protein per kg body weight per day and endurance athletes about 1.2–1.4 g protein per kg body weight per day (to calculate body weight in kg, divide body weight in pounds by 2.2). The protein requirement for nonathletic adults is 0.75 g per kg body weight per day. Protein intakes that would normally promote positive nitrogen balance when energy intake is adequate are not sufficient if energy intake is restricted. This can result in a negative nitrogen balance. Repeated attempts to make weight throughout a season could compromise protein metabolism and thus adversely affect performance.

- *Micronutrients*—intake of minerals and vitamins may be less than optimal, though there may be no visual signs of deficiency. Iron and calcium intakes are often low in female athletes because of poor food choices, avoidance of iron- and calcium-rich foods, and poor eating habits (irregular meals and heavy reliance on snacking). Restricting food intake even more in order to make weight only exacerbates the situation.

Making Weight: The Dilemma

- A female judoist has managed to get her weight down from 60 kg to 58 kg but wishes to compete in the lightweight category (under 56 kg).

- Her present daily calorie intake is 1,500 calories; her carbohydrate intake is 225 g (60 percent of total energy intake).

- On a weight basis, her carbohydrate intake is 3.9 g per kg body weight per day. This amount of carbohydrate is not enough to replenish muscle glycogen stores on a daily basis.

- She drops her intake to 1,000 calories per day in an attempt to get her weight down to under 56 kg. If she keeps to a carbohydrate intake of 60 percent of total energy, it will provide only 2.6 g carbohydrate per kg body weight per day.

- If she attempts to train hard in order to keep up the weight loss, she may end up at the competition "dead at the weight."

Case Study: A Lightweight Female Rower

- J.B. started rowing when she was 18. She was a skinny girl, not at all worried about weight. Two years later she became a vegetarian, much more aware of what she was eating. Four years later J.B. participated in her first year of rowing lightweight. It was her first time on the team and training was hard. The weight dropped off easily and she came

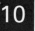
down from 60 kg to 57 kg. In fact, she had to eat a lot to hold her weight at 57 kg. During the winter, her weight increased to 62 kg, 2 kg more than she had ever weighed before. The next season, J.B. was asked to reduce her weight to 56 kg. She cut down the amount of food she was eating, cut out fat, and stopped drinking alcohol. She made weight by diet alone—no sweating—and managed to keep this weight throughout the racing season. After a successful world championship, her weight went up to 65 kg in the winter as she enjoyed a "normal life." Then the dieting season started again, and J.B. had to get down to 56 kg, though at the last minute she was allowed to weigh in at 57 kg. This time, however, she had to sweat to get to 57 kg.

- For the worlds, J.B. had to get down to 56 kg—by calorie counting, cutting back on carbohydrates, and eating lots of vegetables and prepackaged meals of known caloric content. J.B. was now taking 15–20 laxatives a day, doing sweat paddles, and even contemplating cutting her hair to help her get to weight. She felt weak and shaky at the worlds and did not do well.

- The next winter her weight went up to 69 kg and by Easter it was still at 67 kg. J.B.'s diet was no more than 1,200 calories; Diet Cokes figured in very prominently as a way of filling up on no calories. Her weight went down to 63 kg and then stabilized. Next came the rhubarb diet (the food with the lowest calorific value) and more laxatives.

- At this stage, J.B. enlisted the help of a sports dietitian who immediately put her on a 1,500-calorie diet with a high carbohydrate content and changed her eating habits to maximize refueling post-training. J.B. made 59 kg at the worlds without the use of laxatives or sweating, and she and the rest of the crew came back with the silver medal.

What Are the Problems Caused by Dehydration?

A weight loss of as little as 2 percent of body weight can impair performance. Body water is found predominantly in lean tissue—muscles, blood, and vital organs—rather than in body fat tissue. Dehydration by any method leads to a fall in plasma volume, which in turn can lead to a fall in cardiac output, a rise in heart rate, and a fall in blood pressure. It can also contribute to a drop in blood flow to the kidneys, skin, and muscles. As the body becomes more dehydrated, the ability to produce sweat declines, and the temperature-regulation mechanism is compromised. Prolonged exercise or heat exposure in a dehydrated state can ultimately result in heat exhaustion or heat stroke.

Diuretics cause a greater loss of fluid from the circulation than any other method of dehydration. They also promote a loss of sodium and chloride from the blood and potassium and magnesium from muscle cells. A combined loss of minerals and water increases the risk of muscle cramps and spasms. The use of diuretics is not recommended: indeed, the IOC has added diuretics to the list of drugs banned for use by athletes in Olympic competition. Many other governing bodies also ban them.

Dehydration does not affect muscle glycogen stores unless the dehydration is achieved by undergoing strenuous exercise to increase sweat losses. However, when dehydration is accompanied by restricted food intake, the body's total water content and muscle glycogen stores will both be depleted.

What Effects Can Rapid Weight Loss Have on Performance?

Rapid weight loss has a profound adverse effect on aerobic performance. There is conflicting evidence, however, from studies of the effects particularly of dehydration, of making weight on "high-power" performance. Dehydration does not appear to adversely affect performance that lasts less than 30 seconds. However, the ability to sustain near maximal efforts for more than 30 seconds may be reduced.

Finally, rapid weight loss can cause mood changes that have a negative influence on performance; and the general symptoms associated with starvation—tiredness, nausea, and dizziness—can be very detrimental.

Is There a Health Hazard to Yo-Yo Dieting?

Yo-yo dieting is the term used to describe repeated cycles of weight loss and weight gain. A very restricted calorie diet is usually followed, producing an initial weight loss. The diet is often difficult to follow, however, and certainly hard to maintain. Thus, it is eventually abandoned and the weight returns (often with more in addition). The cycle is then repeated, but each time the dieter finds it harder and harder to maintain the weight loss.

Until recently, the accepted explanation for this phenomenon was that the metabolic rate falls during the dieting period as the body adapts to a state of semistarvation and learns to survive on fewer calories. This lower metabolic rate was thought to be maintained after dieting stopped so that, in effect, fewer calories were needed to maintain weight. A return to the predieting calorie intake would therefore result in further weight increases.

That theory is now being questioned. Research carried out at the Medical Research Council's Dunn Nutrition Unit in Cambridge, England, shows that, while metabolism is certainly suppressed when one diets, the metabolic rate bounces back up again when the diet is stopped. Researchers at the Dunn found that after three yo-yo cycles the metabolic rate was exactly the same as when the group of dieters started—*and* they were 12 pounds lighter. Therefore, it would seem that regular dieting does not permanently damage metabolism.

The emotional strain and sheer frustration of yo-yo dieting might explain why many people resist progressive attempts to lose weight. Women in the Cambridge study admitted that they were fed up with the diet by the time the third dieting phase came, and they certainly cheated more during the last diet cycle. Yo-yo dieting seems to be more of a problem if a rapid weight-loss method such as a very restricted calorie diet is used. There is also some concern that in the long term, weight cycling may lead to certain health risks, such as an increase in coronary heart disease and high blood pressure.

How Can I Make Weight Safely?

There are three areas to be considered when planning a program to make weight. First, body weight should be controlled in the off-season, so that the amount of weight that must be lost during the training phase and the run-up to competition can be achieved without severe calorie restrictions or anything more than a minimal weight loss by dehydration. Second, the coach and the athlete should agree on a realistic competition weight. Third, weight loss should be gradual and achieved by using sound nutritional practices to ensure an increase in the ratio of lean body mass to body fat.

How Can I Control My Off-Season Weight?

Table 10.1: *Typical Example of Weight Ranges for a Lightweight Female Rower*

Competition weight	57 kg (125 lbs.)
Training weight	57–60 kg (125–132 lbs.)
Living weight	60–62 kg (132–136 lbs.)

Every athlete has a "living" weight range, a "training" weight range, and a realistic competition weight. The weight ranges differ from individual to individual.

Athletes who have to control their weight during the competition season may like to "live normally" during the "down" period between the end of a season and the start of the next season's program. They eat and drink without restriction, snack, eat meals, and enjoy foods they deny themselves all season. The more weight they put on, however, the more weight they will have to lose once training begins. During the down period, many athletes don't bother to even weigh themselves, and so have no way of knowing the extent of their weight gain. It is a good idea, in such cases, for the athlete to both set an upper limit to the "living" weight range and do weekly weighings, in order to curtail excessive weight gains.

How Can I Decide on a Competition Weight?

To determine your weight category for a new season, enlist the help of a qualified sports dietitian or nutritionist who can estimate your minimal weight by measuring your body fat and calculating how much fat you can afford to lose without affecting health or performance. The actual amount of weight you can afford to lose is calculated by subtracting your minimal weight from your present weight. This calculation should help you to determine your realistic weight category. As a general guide, if you always have to lose 5 kg (11 lbs.) or more to make weight, you should reconsider the weight category you are competing in.

How Should the Weight Loss Be Achieved?

A well-planned dietary strategy should enable you to lose slowly and steadily while still maintaining your training program. You should aim for a maximum weekly weight loss of 0.5–1.0 kg (1 to 2 lbs.). Ideally, you should reach your competition weight between 3 and 5 days before you have to weigh in. Certainly you should be very close to weight 2 or 3 days prior to the competition, with nothing left to do but a little fine tuning.

To achieve a weight loss of 0.5 kg per week, there must be a weekly deficit of 3,500 calories. Daily calorie deficits therefore need to be 500–1,000 calories. The overall intake should never fall below 1,200 calories per day, and during more intensive phases of your training program you will need to increase to 1,500 or even 1,800 calories per day if you are going to refuel effectively after each training session. Be guided by your weekly weight loss and by how your training is going as to whether you are achieving the right intake. Too rapid a weight loss means you need to increase your intake; no weight loss over 2 weeks means you need to cut back more.

The carbohydrate intake should be as high as possible to promote glycogen synthesis. A high proportion of starchy carbohydrate foods should be included to add bulk to the diet. Fat content needs to be reduced to a maximum of 25 percent of total energy, and protein needs to be maintained at a minimum of 15 percent of total energy. It is important to select foods that are nutrient-dense—low in calories but high in nutritional value—if the requirements of vitamins and minerals are to be met.

So What Should I Eat?

The emphasis of your diet should be on bread, pasta, rice, potatoes (baked or boiled), breakfast cereals (preferably fortified with iron), legumes (peas, beans, lentils), fruits and fruit juices, and vegetables. You should also include low-fat dairy foods—such as skim or low-fat milk, yogurts, and cheeses (cottage cheese, low-fat soft cheese)—to ensure an adequate intake of calcium. If you eat meat, include some lean red meat to help maintain your iron intake, but also include chicken (skinless) and fish. Vegetarians should include legumes, soy products, and eggs to ensure a good intake of protein. Cheese is a good source of protein, but most varieties also have high fat contents. To boost iron intake, try to have a bowl of iron-fortified breakfast cereal with low-fat milk and a glass of orange juice. The vitamin C in the juice helps the body to absorb the iron in the cereal, which is otherwise not very well absorbed. Include a variety of vegetables, particularly broccoli, spinach, green peppers, tomatoes, and carrots, as well as lots of fruit. Fruit and vegetables tend to be low in calories yet provide a range of vitamins in reasonable amounts.

Because your intake of vitamins will probably decrease with decreasing calorie intake, it is a good idea to take a multivitamin supplement with iron on a daily basis, if only as an insurance policy. However, it is important that you choose the correct type. You need to buy a supplement that gives you 100 percent of the RDAs (Recommended Dietary Allowances) and no more. There is no benefit from taking megadoses of vitamins.

══Practical Points══

- If you still need to lose weight in the last 7 to 10 days before an event, reduce your energy intake slightly (especially if you are tapering down). However, you need to maintain your intake of carbohydrates, so be even stricter with the fats: use no fat on bread (e.g., butter, mayonnaise); drink skim milk only.

- Reduce your salt intake by not adding salt at the table or in cooking and by avoiding high-salt foods (many of which are high in fat as well).

- Eat a low-fiber diet for the last 24 hours—switch to white bread, low-fiber breakfast cereals, etc.

- After weigh-in, start rehydrating as soon as possible if you have had to do any last minute dehydrating. How effective this will be depends on the amount of body weight lost through dehydration and the time you have between weighing-in and competing. What to drink? Having plain water makes you feel less thirsty and less inclined to drink; it also stimulates urine production. Both of these factors will delay the rehydration process. By contrast, a drink containing some electrolytes (particularly sodium), some carbohydrate, and some water will help you to rehydrate efficiently. Isotonic sports drinks such as Isostar and Gatorade are suitable.

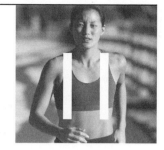

Eating Plans and Snacks

Anita Bean, B.Sc., and Peggy Wellington, B.Sc. (Hons), M.Phil.

Eating Plans

The following plans have been carefully formulated to help you balance and regulate your daily nutritional intake.

Sample Eating Plan Providing Approximately 2,000 Calories

Breakfast: 50 g (2 oz.) whole-grain breakfast cereal
150 ml (1/4 pint) skim/low-fat milk
1 banana

Snack: 1 apple
1 low-fat yogurt

Lunch: 225 g (8 oz.) baked potato
1 tsp. (5 ml) low-fat spread
100 g (4 oz.) tuna mixed with 100 g (4 oz.)
low-fat cottage cheese
1 low-fat yogurt
1 orange

Snack: 1 English muffin with low-fat spread

Dinner: 200 g (7 oz.) chicken leg, grilled and
skinned
or 200 g (7 oz.) cooked legumes
tomato salad with herbs
green salad with 1 tbsp. (15 ml) olive oil/
vinegar dressing
75 g (3 oz.) rice (uncooked weight)
175 g (6 oz.) fruit salad

Nutritional information:

Energy: 2,026 calories; carbohydrate: 318 g (63 percent of calories); fat: 38 g (17 percent of calories); protein: 103 g (20 percent of calories)

Sample Eating Plan Providing Approximately 2,500 Calories

Breakfast: 75 g (3 oz.) whole-grain breakfast cereal
150 ml (¼ pint) skim/low-fat milk
150 ml (¼ pint) fruit juice
1 slice toast with low-fat spread and honey
   or jam

Snack: 1 mini pita filled with 50 g (2 oz.) cottage
   cheese
100 g (4 oz.) grapes/plums/apricots

Lunch: 1 large whole-meal roll with low-fat spread
1 hard-boiled egg with lettuce and tomato
   or 75 g (3 oz.) chicken with lettuce and tomato
1 low-fat yogurt
1 banana

Snack: 1 fruit scone with jam or fruit spread

Dinner: 100 g (4 oz.) pasta (uncooked weight)
100 g (4 oz.) Neopolitan sauce mixed with
   75 g (3 oz.) lean ground beef, ground
   turkey, or cooked lentils
225 g (8 oz.) vegetables or salad
225 g (8 oz.) rice pudding
100 g (4 oz.) fruit (e.g., apricots, pineapple)

Snack: 3 whole-meal crackers
25 g (1 oz.) hard cheese

Nutritional information:

Energy: 2,640 calories; carbohydrate: 433 g (66 percent of calories); fat: 56 g (19 percent of calories); protein: 103 g (16 percent of calories)

Sample Eating Plan Providing Approximately 3,000 Calories

Breakfast:
75 g (3 oz.) whole-grain breakfast cereal
300 ml (½ pint) skim/low-fat milk
150 ml (¼ pint) fruit juice
2 slices toast with low-fat spread and
   honey or jam

Snack:
2 slices whole-meal bread with 50 g
   (2 oz.) tuna or cottage cheese
2 apples (or other fruit)

Lunch:
225 g (8 oz.) baked potato with low-fat
   spread
175 g (6 oz.) baked beans
1 low-fat yogurt
1 orange (or other fruit)

Snack:
1 bagel with low-fat spread

Dinner:
75 g (3 oz.) pasta (uncooked weight)
1 tbsp. olive oil
175 g (6 oz.) white fish or cooked
   lentils/beans
225 g (8 oz.) vegetables or salad
approx. 4 heaped tbsp. fruit crumble
150 ml (¼ pint) custard made with low-fat
   milk

Snack:
1 slice toast with low-fat spread
1 banana

Nutritional information:

Energy: 3,227 calories; carbohydrate: 530 g (66 percent of calories); fat: 63 g (18 percent of calories); protein: 135 g (17 percent of calories)

Snack Attack!

Here are some easy-to-make, high-carbohydrate, low-fat snacks. They are ideal for women on the run since they can be made in bulk and frozen or stored for several days.

Speedy Apple and Cranberry Muffins
12 servings

265 g (9 oz.) self-rising flour (white or whole-meal)

75 g (3 oz.) brown sugar

1 egg

185 ml (¾ cup) skim milk

3 tbsp. melted butter or margarine

80 g (3½ oz.) cranberry sauce

80 g (3½ oz.) applesauce

Mix flour and sugar in a large bowl. Beat egg and stir into flour and sugar. Add milk and melted butter and mix well. Divide mixture into lightly greased muffin tins. Bake at 350° for 20–25 minutes or until golden brown.

Nutritional information (per muffin):

Energy: 177 calories; carbohydrate: 30 g (68 percent of calories); fat: 5 g (25 percent of calories); protein: 3 g (7 percent of calories); fiber: 1 g

Cheesy Scones

10 servings

375 g (13 oz.) self-rising flour (white or whole-meal)

50 g (2 oz.) grated, reduced-fat cheddar cheese

Grainy mustard

4 tbsp. freshly chopped chives or spring onions

45 g (1½ oz.) low-fat natural yogurt

185 ml (¾ cup) skim milk

Mix flour, cheese, chives, and plenty of black pepper in bowl. Stir in yogurt, milk, and mustard (to taste) to form dough. Knead dough on well-floured board and press into a round about 1¼ inch thick. Cut dough into 2-inch rounds, and place on greased baking tray. Brush tops of scones with milk. Bake at 350° for 12–15 minutes or until brown.

Nutritional information (per scone):

Energy: 158 calories; carbohydrate: 29 g (74 percent of calories); fat: 2 g (11 percent of calories); protein: 6 g (15 percent of calories); fiber: 1 g

Mix and Match Cake

16 servings

375 g (13 oz.) self-rising flour (white or whole-meal)

2 eggs

5 tbsp. sunflower oil

1–2 tsp. vanilla extract

1 tsp. salt

200 g (8 oz.) brown sugar

200 g (8 oz.) raisins

3 large ripe bananas

Mix together sugar, eggs, oil, vanilla, and salt. Stir in mashed bananas and raisins and fold in flour. Pour into a well-greased square cake pan and bake at 350° for 40–45 minutes or until cooked. Slice into 16 servings.

Nutritional information (per slice):

Energy: 251 calories; carbohydrate: 44 g (70 percent of calories); fat: 7 g (25 percent of calories); protein: 3 g (5 percent of calories); fiber: 1 g

To mix and match, replace the raisins and bananas above with 200 g each of:

> canned peaches or pineapple (well-drained) and grated carrot
>
> *or* applesauce and chopped dates
>
> *or* cranberry sauce and chopped apricots
>
> *or* plain or flavored yogurt and fresh or frozen strawberries.

Fruit Salad Loaf

12 servings

375 g (13 oz.) self-rising flour (white or whole-meal)

100 g (4 oz.) chopped dried apricots

100 ml (¼ cup plus 2 tbsp.) orange juice

2 apples, grated

1 large ripe banana

1 egg

150 g (6 oz.) sugar

50 g (2 oz.) butter

Combine sugar, butter, apricots, and orange juice in a saucepan. Heat (without boiling) until the sugar has dissolved. Pour into a large bowl and add apple, banana, and beaten egg. Sift the flour and fold into the mixture. Pour into a greased loaf pan and bake at 350° for 40–45 minutes or until cooked.

Nutritional information (per slice):

Energy: 228 calories; carbohydrate: 44 g (77 percent of calories); fat: 4 g (16 percent of calories); protein: 4 g (7 percent of calories); fiber: 2 g

Index

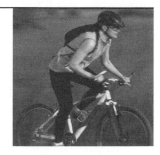

runners, 64; and bone density, 70–72; and eating disorders, 128; and sports anemia, 52–54

S

sailing, 64
salmonella, 40
scones, 172
selenium, 22
sex hormones, 69–73
sex-specific fat, 12
skaters, 64; and eating disorders, 128
skiing, 64
snacks, frequency, 8, 113; recipes, 171–174
soccer, 80, 81, 84
softball, 83
soy, glycemic index, 9
Speedy Apple and Cranberry Muffins, 171
sports anemia, 52–58; causes, 52–54; symptoms, 50; treatment, 56–58
sports drinks, 85–86, 148, 151, 152
sports performance, and low body mass, 64
stress fractures, 73–74
stress, 68
sugar, and iron absorption, 48
surfing, 64
swimming, 64

T

tea, and iron absorption, 48
team sports, carbohydrate recommendations for, 82–83; dietary recommendations for, 81; eating disorders, 82, 128; game preparation, 84–86; long-term nutrition strategies for, 83–84; low energy intake, 81–82; nutrition for, 79–88; player eating habits, 80–81; short-term nutrition strategies for, 84
teenagers, nutrition for, 16–21
tendon injuries, 73
thiamine, recommended intake of, 14; during pregnancy, 34
thinness, obsession with, 118
tofu, protein content, 11
training volume, 66
triathlon, 64

V

vegetables, glycemic index, 9; iron content, 51
vegetarianism, 64, 67
vitamin A, 13; during pregnancy, 34, 38–39; recommended intake, 14
vitamin B12, during pregnancy, 34; recommended intake, 14, 15
vitamin B6, during pregnancy, 34; recommended intake, 14, 15
vitamin C, iron absorption, 48; during pregnancy, 34; recommended intake, 14; sources of, 23, 37
vitamin D, 13; foods containing, 37
vitamin E, 13; sources, 23
vitamin K, 13
vitamin needs during pregnancy, 33
vitamin supplements, 13–16; older athletes and, 22–23
VO$_2$ max (maximum aerobic capacity), 42, 56; reduction of in dieting, 122
vomiting, 124, 158

W

walking, 64
water polo, 64
weight gain during pregnancy, 28–30, 31
weight loss, 89–104; children and teenagers, 18, 19–20; effects on performance, 162; strategies, 105–115
weight-bearing exercise, 102
weight-class sports, nutrition for, 144–145, 157–166
weightlifting, 64
windsurfing, 64
work rates, team sports, 80
workouts, eating for, 8–9
wrestling, 64

Y

yogurt, protein content, 11
yo-yo dieting, hazards, 163

Z

zinc, foods containing, 37; needs during pregnancy, 35; recommended intake, 14, 22

THE COMPLETE GUIDE TO JOSEPH H. PILATES' TECHNIQUES OF PHYSICAL CONDITIONING

Applying the Principles of Body Control

by Allen Menezes, Founder of the Pilates Institute of Australasia

Almost 80 years ago, Joseph Pilates developed a bodywork system that is wildly popular today. Initially taken up by dancers and performers, his program focused on strengthening the core muscles of the abdomen and strengthening and increasing flexibility in the arms and legs. Today his techniques are practiced by celebrities such as Madonna, Vanessa Williams, Patrick Swayze, and Leonardo DiCaprio to maintain a sculpted but not overly muscular look.

Allan Menezes's guide to Joseph Pilates' techniques includes a complete floor program (no special equipment needed) that guides readers through basic, intermediate, and advanced routines, with detailed descriptions of each exercise and step-by-step photographs. There is a special section on relieving back, ankle, and shoulder pain, and insights on how the work can be adapted by athletes. Worksheets are provided to record progress, and an introduction gives the history and legacy of Joseph Pilates.

Comprehensive and precise, this book is for those who make feeling healthy and looking fit a way of life. Everyone—from

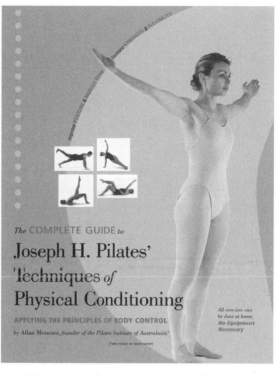

208 pages ... 191 b/w photos ... 80 illus. & charts
Paperback $19.95 ... Spiral Bound $26.95

new mothers to ballet dancers, from those with lower back pain to those who simply wish to improve their strength and flexibility—will benefit from this book.

Allen Menezes is the founder of the Pilates Institute of Australasia and the Body Control Pilates Australia exercise studio franchise. He lectures internationally and conducts workshops and intensive instructor trainer courses for laypeople as well as healthcare professionals.

***To order, or for our FREE catalog of books, please see last page
or call 1-800-266-5592. Prices subject to change.***

GET FIT WHILE YOU SIT

Easy Workouts from Your Chair

by Charlene Torkelson

Get Fit While You Sit is a total body workout that can be done right from your chair, anywhere. It's perfect for office workers, travelers, and those with age-related movement limitations or special conditions. There are no complicated routines, no expensive gym memberships, and no pieces of equipment requiring a lot of space. You can even build these chair exercises into your daily home or office routine.

The book offers three carefully designed programs. **The One-Hour Chair Program** is a full-body, low-impact workout that includes light aerobics and isolation exercises to be done with or without weights. A section highlights exercises for problem areas such as the back, upper legs, and stomach, and special conditions including arthritis and osteoporosis. **The Five-Day Short Program** features five complete, compact workouts for those short on time. Finally, computer users, travelers, and the truly rushed will enjoy the **Ten-Minute Miracles,** a group of easy-to-do exercises perfect for anyone at the office—even in a meeting or on the go.

Each section includes clear directions and step-by-step photographs, and there is a checklist for monitoring progress. Written in a clear, encouraging, upbeat style, this is

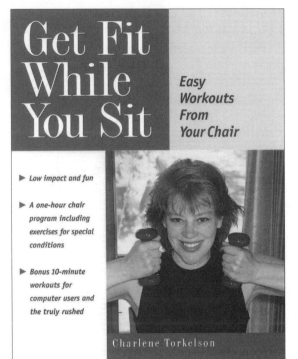

160 pages ... 212 b/w photos
Paperback $12.95 ... Spiral Bound $17.95
Hard Cover $22.95

one program you'll stick with even if you've given up on others. No time? No space? No excuses—just get fit while you sit!

Charlene Torkelson has been a dance and exercise expert for more than twenty years. She currently teaches a popular "chair class," and lives in Golden Valley, Minnesota, with her husband and three young children.

TREAT YOUR BACK WITHOUT SURGERY

The Best Non-Surgical Alternatives for Eliminating Back and Neck Pain

by Stephen Hochschuler, M.D., and Bob Reznik, MBA

In this easy-to-read guide to back care and early treatment the authors—experts in the field—present non-surgical options for treating back pain, including:

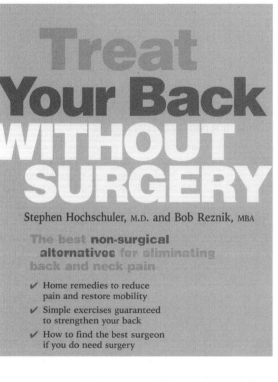

- The four steps of first aid (ice, then heat—take anti-inflammatories—rest, but only for 2 days—as soon as you can, walk)

- an illustrated program of exercises that make the back muscles stronger and more flexible

- non-invasive treatments such as manipulation, physical therapy, and chiropractic

- alternative therapies like acupuncture, magnetic therapy, and tai chi

224 pages ... 47 b/w photos ... 6 illus.
Paperback $14.95
Hard cover $24.95

According to the authors, "virtually any non-surgical treatment that will not make you worse may be worth a try before you resort to surgery." Recognizing that surgery may be necessary at times, however, they offer guidelines on what to expect from diagnostic tests, how each type of surgery works, what kind of surgeon to choose, and how to find a good spine treatment center.

Stephen Hochschuler is a board-certified orthopedic surgeon specializing in spine surgery, co-founder and chairman of the Texas Back Institute, and co-author of *Back in Shape*. Bob Reznik helped develop the Texas Back Institute Back Pain Hotline and currently runs Prizm Development, a company that works with healthcare providers to develop consumer-friendly centers of excellence.

To order, or for our FREE catalog of books, please see last page or call 1-800-266-5592. Prices subject to change.

ORDER FORM

10%	DISCOUNT on orders of $50 or more —
20%	DISCOUNT on orders of $150 or more —
30%	DISCOUNT on orders of $500 or more —

On cost of books for fully prepaid orders

NAME

ADDRESS

CITY/STATE   ZIP/POSTCODE

PHONE   COUNTRY (outside of U.S.)

TITLE	QTY	PRICE	TOTAL
Sports Nutrition for Women (paperback)		@ $15.95	
Sports Nutrition for Women (hard cover)		@ $25.95	

Prices subject to change without notice

Please list other titles below:

		@ $	
		@ $	
		@ $	
		@ $	
		@ $	
		@ $	
		@ $	

Check here to receive our book catalog ☐   FREE

Shipping Costs:
First book: $3.00 by book post ($4.50 by UPS, Priority Mail, or to ship outside the U.S.)
Each additional book: $1.00
For rush orders and bulk shipments call us at (800) 266-5592

TOTAL	
Less discount @_____%	( )
TOTAL COST OF BOOKS	_____
Calif. residents add sales tax	_____
Shipping & handling	_____
TOTAL ENCLOSED	_____

Please pay in U.S. funds only

☐ Check ☐ Money Order ☐ Visa ☐ MasterCard ☐ Discover

Card # _____ Exp. date_____

Signature _____

Complete and mail to:
Hunter House Inc., Publishers
PO Box 2914, Alameda CA 94501-0914
Orders: (800) 266-5592 email: ordering@hunterhouse.com
Phone (510) 865-5282 Fax (510) 865-4295
☐ Check here to receive our book catalog

SNW 10/01